John Snow and the Cholera Epidemic of 1854: The History of the Outbreak and Its Impact on Public Health Measures

By Charles River Editors

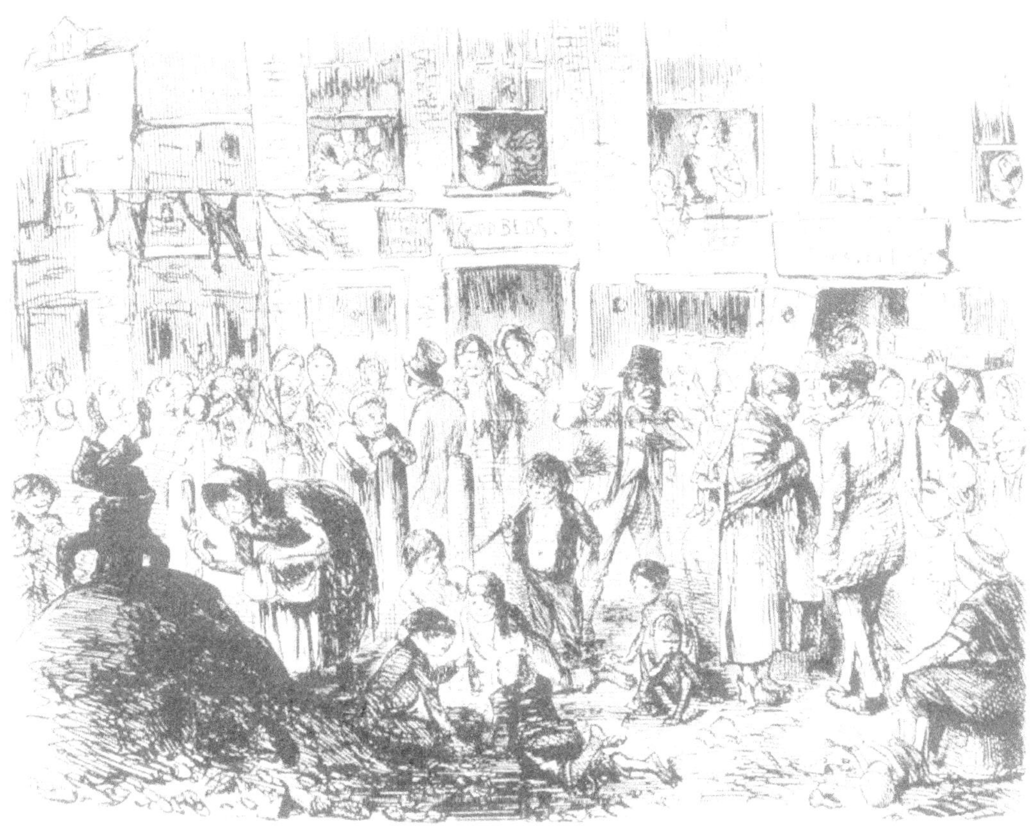

A *Punch* magazine cartoon about the outbreak

About Charles River Editors

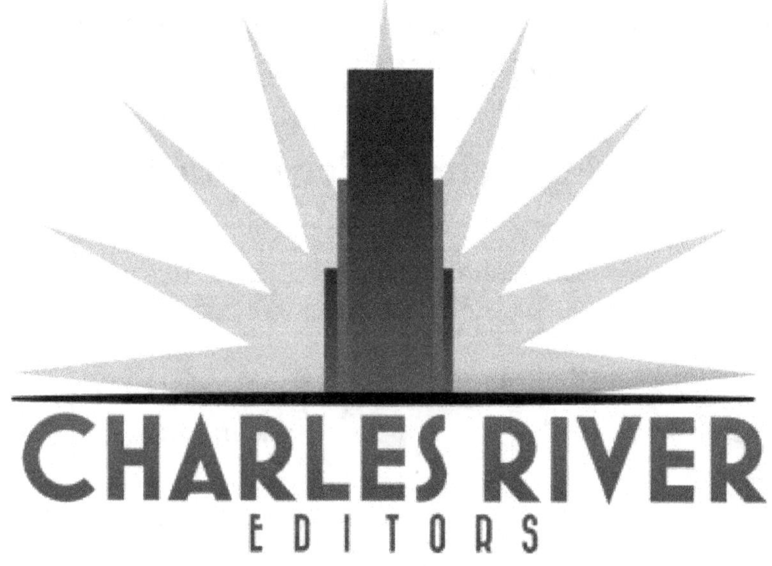

Charles River Editors provides superior editing and original writing services across the digital publishing industry, with the expertise to create digital content for publishers across a vast range of subject matter. In addition to providing original digital content for third party publishers, we also republish civilization's greatest literary works, bringing them to new generations of readers via ebooks.

Sign up here to receive updates about free books as we publish them, and visit Our Kindle Author Page to browse today's free promotions and our most recently published Kindle titles.

Introduction

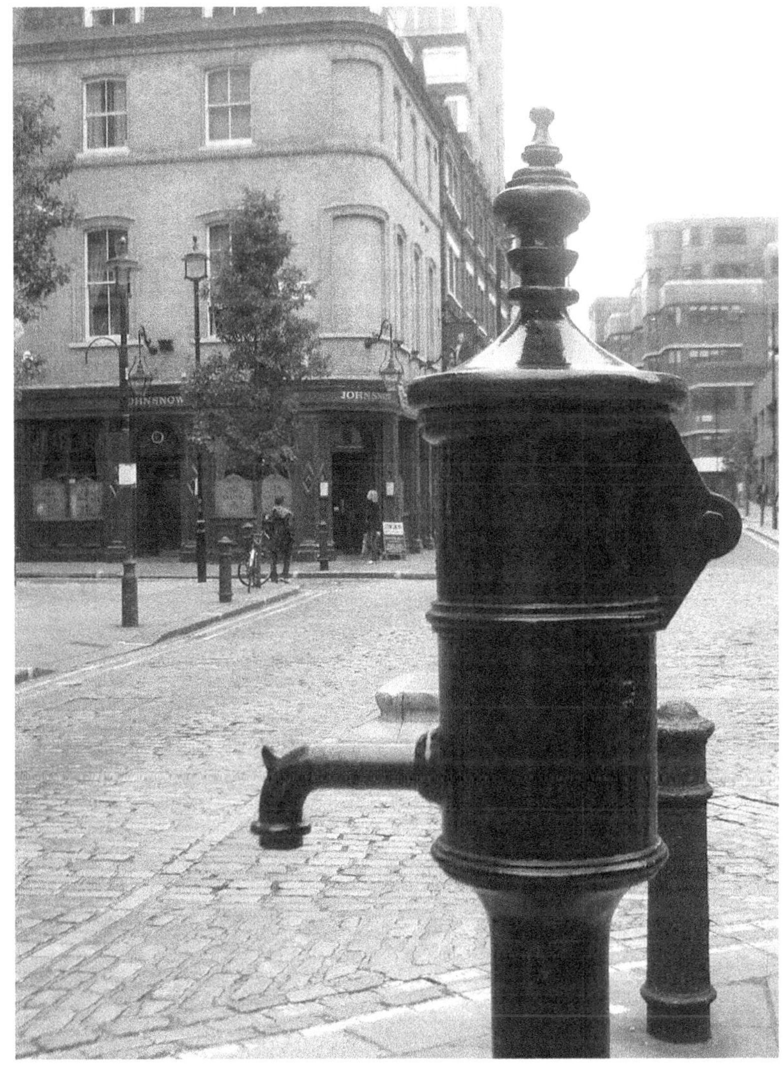

A picture of the John Snow memorial in London

"In many cases a single house has a supply different from that on either side. Each company supplies both rich and poor, both large houses and small; there is no difference in the condition or occupation of the persons receiving the water of the different companies...As there is no difference whatever either in the houses or the people receiving the supply of the two Water Companies, or in

any of the physical conditions with which they are surrounded, it is obvious that no experiment could have been devised which would more thoroughly test the effect of water supply on the progress of Cholera than this, which circumstances placed ready made before the observer. The experiment too, was on the grandest scale. No fewer than three hundred thousand people of both sexes, of every age and occupation, and of every rank and station, from gentlefolks down to the very poor, were divided into two groups without their choice, and, in most cases, without their knowledge; one group being supplied water containing the sewage of London, and amongst it, whatever might have come from the cholera patients, the other group having water quite free from such impurity."
– John Snow

Plague and pestilence have both fascinated and terrified humanity from the very beginning. Societies and individuals have struggled to make sense of them, and more importantly they've often struggled to avoid them. Before the scientific age, people had no knowledge of the microbiological agents – unseen bacteria and viruses – which afflicted them, and thus the maladies were often ascribed to wrathful supernatural forces. Even when advances in knowledge posited natural causes for epidemics and pandemics, medicine struggled to deal with them, and for hundreds of years religion continued to work hand-in-hand with medicine.

Inevitably, that meant physicians tried a variety of practices to cure the sick, and many of them seem quite odd by modern standards. By the time Rome was on the rise, physicians understood that contagions arose and spread, but according to Galen, Hippocrates, and other Greco-Roman authorities, pestilence was caused by *miasma*, foul air produced by the decomposition of organic matter. Though modern scientists have since been able to disprove this, on the face of it there was some logic to the idea. Physicians and philosophers (they were very often the same, Galen being an example) noticed that disease arose in areas of poor sanitation, where filth and rotting matter was prevalent and not disposed of, and the basic measures to prevent disease – waste removal, provision of clean food and water and quarantining - would have been obvious to them. The scenting of miasmic air with incense and other unguents to expel the foulness would also have thus made sense, though people now know that can't stop the spread of a disease.

Even today, potent and adaptive pathogens can leave a wake of high mortality throughout major continents, and recent generations have felt powerless to prevent the onslaught when unfamiliar bacterial or viral populations reach a tipping point and find an opportunity for an incursion into human society. For centuries, the evolution of medical science failed to break through on the microscopic and molecular level to gain insights into the prevention and cure of a specific set of afflictions. These mysterious entities have accompanied people from the beginning, and societies both anticipated and dreaded their unscheduled return. In the mid-19th century, the barrier to understanding the mechanics of such attacks was the failure to pinpoint the vehicles by which the world's preeminent diseases are conveyed to the human race.

In the case of cholera, once among the most dreaded diseases, a breakthrough in Victorian England occurred in the mid-19th century during one of several epidemics to assault the island. In that instance, an unassuming physician named John Snow was able to trace the environmental component in which cholera was carried. He accomplished this in large part through a painstaking map cross-referencing location and specific cases of infection within a small area of London. Eventually, he narrowed the source down to a single manual water pump in the midst of the poverty-stricken neighborhood of Soho.

An extensive early education provided by the first outbreak sent him on a contrarian's path in analyzing the dreaded disease. He was not blessed with the pedigree of an aristocratic family or the attendant gifts required for a young man of social substance to seek a high-level formal education. Nevertheless, he rose to be recognized not only as the world's leading anesthetist, but also as the practitioner who proved that the cholera outbreaks in Britain were the result of polluted water. Today, he is addressed as the "Father of Epidemiology," defined by Webster as a "medical science that deals with the incidence, distribution, and control of disease in a population."[1]

At the time, however, in the face of resistance launched by more powerful and pedigreed members of the medical profession, Snow was rewarded with criticism for not successfully revealing the entirety of the disease's inner mechanics. It was only over the course of several decades that Snow was able to persuade the medical community at large of the disease's source, and the British successfully established policies that helped prevent future outbreaks. Ironically, Snow eventually gained membership in Britain's high circle of elite medical practitioners, but it was not his work on cholera that initially propelled him to global fame. Ultimately, it was his pioneering work in the new field of anesthesiology, largely unknown to Britain, that earned the applause of contemporaries.

John Snow and the Cholera Epidemic of 1854: The History of the Outbreak and Its Impact on Public Health

---

[1] Dale P. Sandler, John Snow and Modern-Day Epidemiology – www.academic.oup.com/aje/article/152/1/1/139141

Measures examines the deadly outbreak and Snow's groundbreaking findings. Along with pictures depicting important people, places, and events, you will learn about the cholera outbreak like never before.

John Snow and the Cholera Epidemic of 1854: The History of the Outbreak and Its Impact on Public Health Measures

Previous Efforts to Fight Outbreaks

The earliest record of any kind of systematized healthcare dates to ancient Mesopotamia and the Sumerian and Babylonian civilizations. For these, healing was in the gift of the gods and physicians operated as their instruments. The goddess Gula ("the great physician") presided over medicine for the ancient Sumerians.[2] Her son Ninazu was also a healer and assisted her. Ninazu was represented holding a rod around which a serpent was wound, and the snake became a recurring symbol of the medical profession that survives to this day.[3] Ninazu was also god of the underworld and so was master both of death and life. Just as the serpent shed its skin and renewed itself, so Ninazu gave deliverance to his supplicants.[4]

For the ancient Egyptians who took up the mantle of Mesopotamian physicians, medicine channelled the power of the gods. It is often noted that ancient Egyptian medicine was advanced for its time and more enlightened in many respects than that of the Middle Ages. Egyptian physicians were aware of the importance of diet; they employed medicines, had a fairly good (though not complete) knowledge of human anatomy, recognized the

---

[2] Joshua J. Mark, "Health Care in Ancient Mesopotamia", *Ancient History Encyclopedia* May 21, 2014. https://www.ancient.eu/article/687/health-care-in-ancient-mesopotamia/.

[3] Even the monotheistic Hebrews made reference to it as a symbol of healing *vide* Numbers 21:6-8.

[4] Ibid.

healing properties of massage and aromatherapy, and performed surgery, including trepanning. A major source of medical knowledge was the practice of embalming and mummification of bodies in preparation for the afterlife, which was performed by priests. Thus, ancient Egyptian priests were also physicians.

The contagions known to have afflicted the ancient Egyptians include smallpox, typhoid, the common cold, tuberculosis, malaria, dysentery and bilharsiasis, a disease spread by contaminated water.[5] To counter these diseases, priests and priestesses invoked such deities as Sekhmet, Serket, Sobek, and Nefertum. However, one aspect of Egyptian priestly medicine may have done much to prevent the spread of pestilence. Ritual purity was very important to the Egyptians, who were obsessed by cleanliness, so much so that a worshipper could not approach his or her god without washing his body as an exterior expression of their interior purity of intention. All filth and decaying matter had to be removed from the sacred places. As a result, these practices may have inadvertently aided in the containment of contagion, and the sacred precincts to which the sick went might have unintentionally operated as quarantine centers.

Perhaps the most persecuted people in Europe over the

---

[5] Joshia J. Mark, "Ancient Egyptian Medicine", *Ancient History Encyclopedia* February 17, 2017. https://www.ancient.eu/Egyptian_Medicine/.

centuries were the Jews, and it was no different during the Black Death. Muisis reported, "In 1349, Jews were seized and put in chains and into prison everywhere, in all the places where they dwelt. The reason for this as a strong suspicions that they planned to destroy the Christians by means of poison, and that they had secretly put poison into wells, springs and rivers so that Christians would drink it. And the common report was that they had done this in various places. For there were some among the Jews who were cunning and learned astrologers and they had forecast the impending mortality from the course of the stars, and this encouraged them to put their evil intention into practice with more confidence and cunning. They also saw by the course of the stars that a religious sect was to be destroyed (and they hoped that this meant the Christians) and that men bearing red crosses would appear (and they were unsure whether this meant their sect would then be destroyed); and they said many other things which it would take too long to relate here."

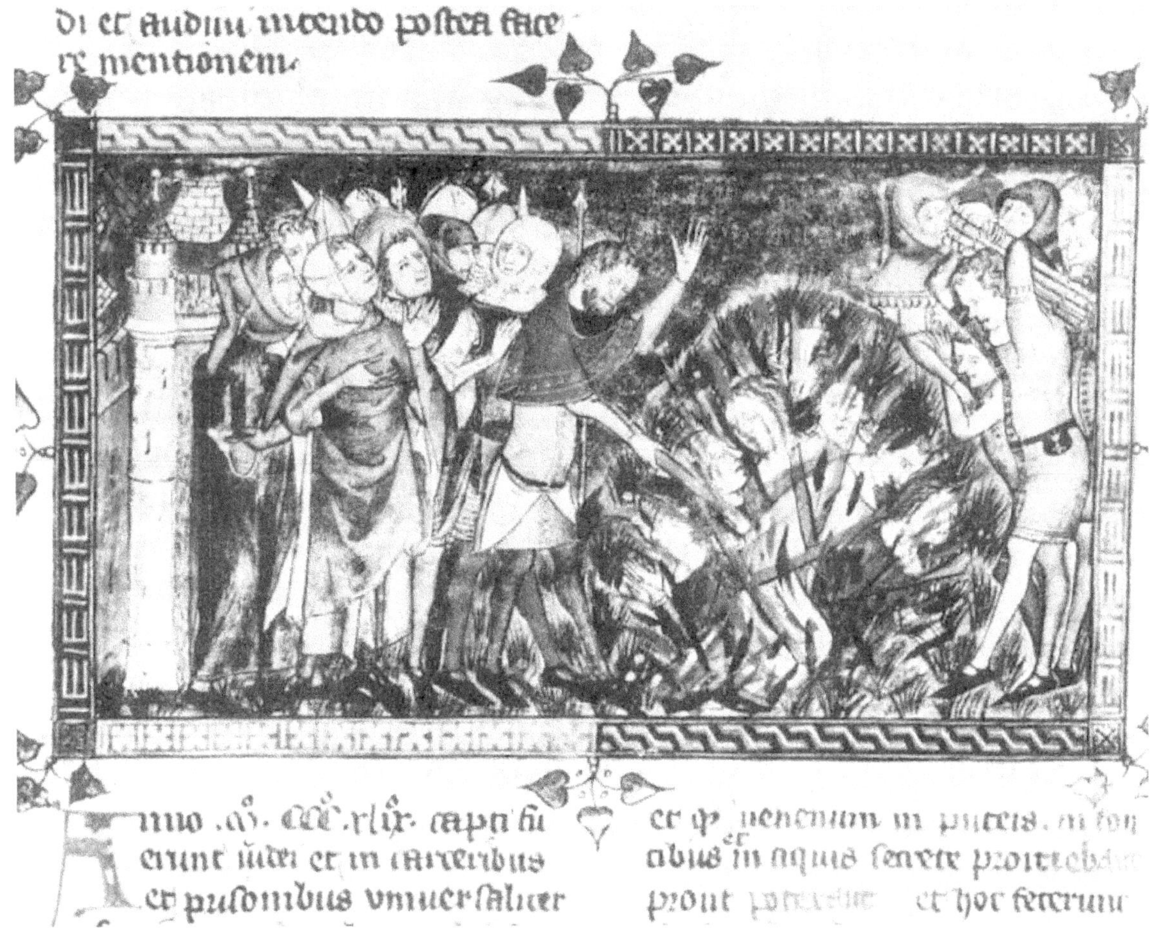

A medieval depiction of Jews being burned in Strasbourg, France

Not only was there an ongoing racial and religious hatred of the people often derisively referred to by Christians as "God's chosen people," but in the case of the Black Death, there seemed to be a rational reason to believe that the Jews were somehow waging a secret war on the Christians. The reason for this assumption was the observation by many that the pestilence did not spread across Jewish communities as much as it did among Gentile ones. What the misled minds did not understand was that the strict dietary and health codes that the Jews observed meant they were living in a much cleaner and healthier environment than their Christian neighbors. Therefore, what seemed to be some sort of conspiracy was actually the result of good hygiene paying off.

In the ancient Greco-Roman world, illness was also seen as divine punishment, though the gods were not perceived as necessarily just. In fact, the gods were believed to be capricious, with personalities and characteristics quite similar to mortals. They could be undependable, avaricious, vainglorious, conceited, vengeful, and vicious, but they were immortal and had powers over humanity that they often used without justice or mercy. In Hebrew and Egyptian theology, there was a standard of morality by which individuals were judged, but not in Greek and Roman theology. Even in death, mortals that offended the gods could be imprisoned in Tartarus, a wasteland of terror and torment below the Earth. It was there that Crete's King Sisyphus eternally rolled a boulder up a mountain, Tantalus was tortured by food and drink he could never reach, and the giant Tityos was torn alive by vultures over and over again. Those beloved by the gods might be placed in the Elysian Fields at the westernmost edge of the Earth, but the common herd of mortals passed eternity in a realm differing little from earthly existence. The evils sent by the gods might be averted by sacrifices, but only for a time, because the wrathful gods might change their minds just as mortals did.

Plagues and pestilence were associated with Apollo, the god of the sun, light, and knowledge. He was revered as a healer, for just as he unleashed plagues he could cause them to cease. An early reference to his might is to found in *The Iliad,* where Homer wrote of the god shooting plague arrows at the Greeks for nine days "with a face as dark as night, and his silver bow rang death as he shot his arrow in the midst of them." Victims of pestilence might visit Apollo's temples and offer sacrifices of expiation.

Asclepius was another god of healing, and he was more approachable than Apollo in that he was more inclined to heal pestilence than inflict it. He was the son of Apollo and a mortal woman named Coronis and thus sympathetic to the plight of weak mortals. He was taught medicine by the centaur Chiron and became a greater healer than even his father. He even learned to raise the dead. Zeus, king of the gods, was so fearful of mortals learning the secret of immortality that he struck Asclepius dead with a thunderbolt. The healer's popularity, however, was so great that Zeus was forced to restore him to life and elevate him to the status of an Olympian god, presumably on the understanding that he would not give the secret of immortality to men.

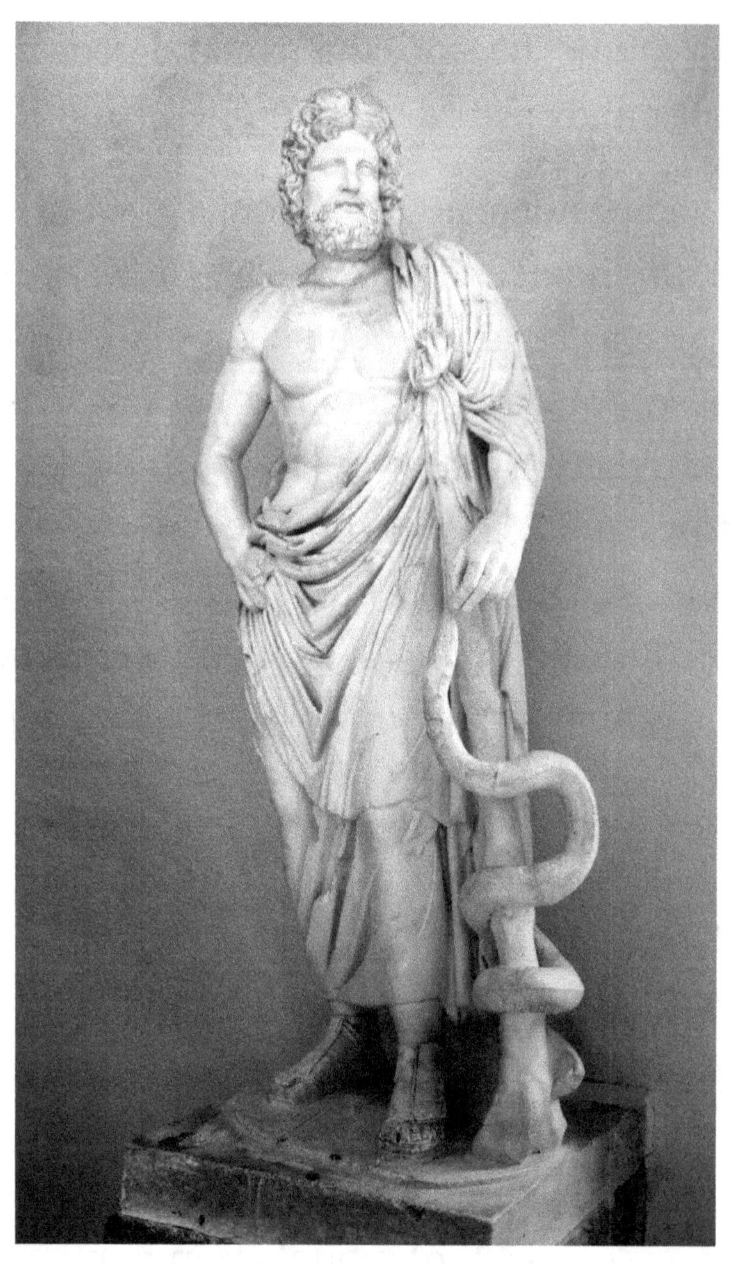

Michael F. Mehnert's picture of an ancient statue of Asclepius

It is probably no coincidence that the cult of Asclepius grew from the 5th century BCE onwards. Plagues broke out in both Italy and Greece in the 430s, and the increased trade between the various Greek colonies scattered about the Mediterranean increased the range of epidemics. Indeed, the first great plagues for which historians have enough material to study date from the period of Hellenic migration. The Plague of Athens, possibly an outbreak of typhus, killed 75,000-100,000 people across Greece from 429-426 BCE.[6] 44 years later, an epidemic – possibly influenza – decimated both the Greek and Italian peninsulas.[7]

The idea that diseases were an affliction from the gods was a powerful one and remains so in some quarters, but 500 years before the elite of the Roman Empire offered coins for the oracles of Glycon, one of the finest minds of the Greek world had already proposed a natural explanation for the morbidities with which humans were afflicted.

Hippocrates, who was born around 460 BCE and died near 370 BCE, was neither a priest nor a prophet, but a physician who had separated medicine from theology. Often called the "Father of Medicine,"[8] Hippocrates held that illness was not a punishment from the gods but the product of factors concerning environment, diet, and behavior.

---

[6] Papagrigorakis, Manolis J.; Yapijakis, Christos; Synodinos, Philippos N.; Baziotopoulou-Valavani, Effie (2007). "DNA examination of ancient dental pulp incriminates typhoid fever as a probable cause of the Plague of Athens". *International Journal of Infectious Diseases*. **10** (3): 206–214.
[7] Potter, C. W. (2002). "Foreword". *Influenza*. Elsevier Science. p. vii.
[8] "Hippocrates". *Microsoft Encarta Online Encyclopedia*. Microsoft Corporation. 2006. Archived from the original on 2009-10-29.

The attitude toward human affliction exhibited by Hippocrates and his students was certainly an advance from sorcery and divine expiation, but his methods were not based on science as people today would understand it. The concept of science as the construction and organization of a body of knowledge based on testable theories simply did not exist at the time.[9] But there was already a rich tradition of philosophy, which differs from science in that it attempts to arrive at knowledge of matter, being, and ethics by rational argument rather than from empirical evidence. The scope of philosophy, which concerns itself with the whole of existence, is much broader than science, which confines its conclusions to the observable world. Therefore, the medicine of Hippocrates would have treated the patient holistically, meaning physically, emotionally, spiritually, and existentially.

Hippocrates and other Greco-Roman physicians were limited by their lack of knowledge of human anatomy because the dissection of corpses was considered disrespectful to the gods who had created humankind, but they believed they knew enough to effectively treat their patients. They held the doctrine of Νόσων φύσεις ἰητροί, or in Latin *Vis medicatrix naturae*, meaning "the healing power of nature." The body possessed the power to heal

---

[9] Lehoux, Daryn (2011). "2. Natural Knowledge in the Classical World". In Shank, Michael; Numbers, Ronald; Harrison, Peter (eds.). *Wrestling with Nature: From Omens to Science*. Chicago: University of Chicago Press. p. 39.

itself and the physician simply aided the patient in his recovery and ensured there were no obstacles. The emphasis was on prognosis rather than diagnosis, for if the body was healing itself, knowing the illness was in a sense unnecessary.[10]

Hippocrates ascribed the spread of contagions to *miasma* (literally, "pollution") or foul air. Miasma was supposed to arise from decaying organic matter and infect its victims as it drifted, and it was identifiable by its noxious smell. The theory had a certain logical coherence since pestilence was observed to break out in locations where there was poor hygiene and sanitation, but it also infected seemingly clean areas. It made sense then to suppose that the rotting matter had befouled the air, which in turn had moved to another location. Physicians urged that outbreaks be prevented by ensuring good sanitation, a measure which no modern medico would disagree with, but the ancient physicians believed that once it had broken out, the air might be purified with sweet-smelling herbs, spices, incense or unguents. This idea persisted both in the West and the East until the latter half of the 19th century, and even today the number of households using "air fresheners" and "purifiers" testifies to its persistence.

Hippocrates believed miasma produced disease in the body by causing an imbalance in its humors. Humorism

---

[10] *Garrison, Fielding H. (1966), History of Medicine, Philadelphia: W.B. Saunders Company*, pp.93–94.

was another medical doctrine of Hippocrates based on philosophy. It rested on the belief of the ancients – notably the Babylonians, Greeks, and the Vedic Indians – that the material elements of the cosmos were air, fire, earth, and water, and that all matter, including the human body, was composed of a balance of the four. The manner in which they balanced might be determined by their properties. Air was hot and wet (as a vapor), fire was hot and dry, earth was cold and dry, and water was of cold and wet. The elements in the body corresponded to four fluids or humors: blood, yellow bile, black bile and phlegm. Blood, being hot and wet, represented air. Yellow bile (the fluid produced by the liver, stored in the gall bladder and sometimes vomited when ill) was supposed to be warm and dry like fire. Black bile (bloody fluid) corresponded to cold and dry earth while phlegm was cold and wet. One's dominant temperament was determined by the balance of fluids and we still use the language of the humors to describe an individual's disposition: sanguine, choleric, melancholic and phlegmatic.

An excess of any of these humors in the body was indicative of an imbalance, and the physician's role was to aid the restoration of balance, so every disease was identified with the excess of a particular humor. In the case of the Antonine Plague, which was probably smallpox, the great Roman physician Galen identified the symptoms with skill and precision, noting erupting ulcers all over the body, the coughing up of *ephelis* (small scabs), and the ulceration of the pharynx, esophagus, and trachea. Modern medicine would recognize these all as clear symptoms of smallpox, and the fact that a physician as educated, skilled, and widely traveled as Galen did not recognize the disease heavily suggests that smallpox was as yet unknown to the Mediterranean world. Galen speculated that the disease was caused by an excess of bile on account of the vomiting of dry blood and the eruption of skin pustules. Bile was considered the most pernicious of the humors,[11] and Galen never arrived at what he might have considered a cure.

In light of the humor theory, Galen's approach to the pestilence hinged on him being able to identify the imbalance of fluids in the bodies of the victims. In other words, he had to determine which humor predominated in those afflicted. Galen wrote extensively about the symptoms of plague victims, but not much about the treatment. The vomiting of dry blood (thought to be bile) and eruption of pustules described by Galen permit the speculation that the disease was caused by an excess of bile, and indeed, bile was considered the most noxious of the humors.[12] Humorist theory held that all the humors

[11] Amir Arsalan Afkhami (2012)"Humoralism" *Encyclopedia Iranica* http://www.iranicaonline.org/articles/humoralism-1
[12] Amir Arsalan Afkhami (2012) "Humoralism"*Encyclopaedia Iranica* http://www.iranicaonline.org/articles/humoralism-1

were present in the blood, so to aid the release of harmful humors, physicians often made an incision to allow blood to drain. This practice, known as bloodletting, was not believed to be dangerous if controlled, as Galen believed that blood was formed in the liver and did not circulate. Despite the fact it didn't work (and often hurt the patient), bloodletting would be practiced well into the 19th century.

Diet was considered the first avenue to restoring the balance of the humors. The adage "you are what you eat" struck especially true for the ancient physician, who believed that certain foods could augment or counter the effects of particular humors. Yellow bile was associated with high temperatures and dryness, black bile with coldness and dryness, phlegm with wet and cold, and blood with heat and moisture. As a result, an excess of black bile might then be treated with foods considered hot, such as garlic, onions, meat and olives.

The emphasis on an appropriate diet probably helped a lot of ill persons, albeit in a somewhat inadvertent and haphazard way. For example, the prescription of only clear, unpolluted water (mountain water was the best)[13] would have not only been beneficial to the patient, but would have assisted in the prevention of contagion, though physicians didn't know the real reasons why.

---

[13] David K. Osborn (2008) "Diet" Food and drink" *Greek Medicine.net*
    http://www.greekmedicine.net/hygiene/Diet_Food_and_Drink.html

Chinese philosophy and medicine were also based on five elements or phases: fire, water, wood, metal, and earth.[14] These were used to explain the body's organs, physical activities, and morbidities. In the 2nd century BCE, elemental theory was incorporated into *Ying-Yan* philosophy, which taught that the cosmos was a whole consisting of contrary but complementary phenomena. As Ying and Yang governed everything, including space and time, the hour at which a patient took a remedy and the place where they took it was often important. A medical journal in 1911 reported a Chinese remedy for the plague: "On the sixth day of the sixth moon gather "Horse Tooth Vegetables" [purslane], dry them in the sun and lay away until New Year's morning, boil until done, and pickle in brine and vinegar for one year. Partaking of this will … prevent the current malady."[15]

Somewhat incredibly, the idea that diseases might be spread by microscopic pathogenic particles was first proposed as far back as the 5th century BCE. The historian Thucydides (c. 460–c. 400 BCE) postulated the existence of spores or *semina* (seeds) that could travel through the air.[16] The Roman scholar Marcus Terrentius Varro (116–27 BCE) went further, coming extraordinarily close to

[14] Dr Zai, J. *Taoism and Science: Cosmology, Evolution, Morality, Health and more*. Ultravisum, 2015.

[15] "Chinese remedies for the plague", *US National Library of Medicine* https://www.ncbi.nlm.nih.gov/pmc/articles/PMC2332311/?page=1.

[16] Singer, Charles and Dorothea (1917) "The scientific position of Girolamo Fracastoro [1478–1553] with especial reference to the source, character and influence of his theory of infection", *Annals of Medical History*, **1**: 1–34.

present knowledge by claiming that "there are bred certain minute creatures which cannot be seen by the eyes, which float in the air and enter the body through the mouth and nose and there cause serious diseases."[17]

Unfortunately, these ideas remained mere speculation and were all but ignored by medicine until the invention of the microscope in the 17th century, and even then the correlation between microscopic organisms and illness was not proved, though there was plenty of speculation. This was still the state of things when a global outbreak of cholera began in the mid-19th century.

John Snow's Background

Cholera was an ancient enemy known to all the world's civilizations. Wherever there was polluted water, outbreaks occurred, from India to Africa and the European continent. Indeed, the term "cholera" can be traced to the Greeks' belief in the four "humours," with cholera being associated with a hot-tempered and easily angered entity. The Greeks set their emphasis on yellow bile, considered to be the predominant "humour" of the summer season. In such a context, cholera was not in itself a disease, but an excessive burgeoning of yellow bile attempting to purge the body of its ills. Although the Greeks could not ultimately solve the riddle at the microscopic level, the

---

[17] Varro, Marcus Terentius with Lloyd Storr-Best, trans., *Varro on Farming* (London, England: G. Bell and Sons, Ltd., 1912), Book 1, Ch. XII, p. 39.

approach was guided by a fair sense of logic, albeit in a highly metaphorical expression. Such an outbreak of "yellow bile" was eventually given the name of *cholera morbus*, or "bile sickness." The original term of *cholera* was the name bestowed upon the affliction by Hippocrates himself.

In other cultures, it went by different names, such as the Arabic word "heyda." Even in that distant past, practitioners noted the appearance of white particles resembling "rice-water like"[18] flecks in the feces of victims.

In the post-Newtonian and Cartesian world, the body began to be viewed as a machine, representative of a parallel vision of the coming Industrial Revolution. Despite the dread brought on by an earlier onset of the Black Death that killed a third of Europe's population, localized and regional outbreaks of cholera troubled Britain at regular intervals in this medically curious new century. The four outbreaks on the island, in 1831, 1848, 1853, and 1866, seemed like a curse upon the lengthy reign of Queen Victoria, who heavily mourned the unexplainable loss of her subjects.

From the earliest outbreak, the self-appointed superiority of British culture laid claim to its own version of the

---

[18] Stephen W. Lacey, Cholera: Calamitous Past, Ominous Future, *Clinical Infectious Diseases* Vol. 20 No. 5 (May 1995)

disease, unwilling to suffer the same variety plaguing lesser realms in exotic locales. Britain was rife with travelers and explorers circling the globe in what has been termed a "free trade of diseases."[19] However, British travel was not typically accused as the culprit; after all, expansion was the watchword of the empire, a healthy expression of its credo: "Britain's way is the world's way." The blame lay rather on an influx of dubious visitors from foreign lands, who were accused of bringing along their various maladies. In the Victorian vision, the presence of *"cholera nostra,"* or "our cholera," stood in direct opposition to the fearsome Asiatic cholera, of which the subtext was "their cholera." In the British worldview, such a disease belonged to a land of "filthy, uncivilized savages"[20] living outside the benefits of British advancement.

However, rather than picking off the weak strays of British societies, Asiatic cholera overwhelmed victims of all ages and types, including the young, old, strong, and weak. Death came quickly from the rapid onset in the majority of cases. Such rapidity was an offense to the British ideal of "a good death," one in which a citizen was given enough time to prepare, to get his or her affairs in order, and to wait in a quietly posed state of dignity. The ruthless ambush of eastern cholera was in all ways

____

[19] Sick City Project
[20] Sick City Project

repugnant to the Victorian vision.

It was in addressing these realities that medical experts ran into another British bias. Poverty was not a mere economic condition in the epicenter of the empire, but an outright moral failing. Indiscriminate to human concerns as the disease was, it nevertheless found the greatest abundance of opportunities among the poor, who were generally less able to mount a defense. The prevailing analysis of the time described cholera as an environmental toxin originating and traveling by air in clouds of generic, polluted vapors, but even the most decorated physicians and surgeons took far too long in recognizing that the disease was never to be found in the nose or lungs. Rather, in every case, the affliction was an intestinal disorder. Once that reality became undeniable, the prevailing theory adjusted itself to a belief that cholera entered the respiratory system before leaping to the digestive. It was a neat answer that eliminated the need for a paradigm shift that might require saving face, and thus, little mention was made of a total absence of residual disease in the nostrils and airways by which it allegedly entered.

Cholera's first symptom was usually queasiness, followed by sudden vomiting and diarrhea. In such a sudden onset, a dramatic state of dehydration was typical, followed by a general circulatory collapse. In a death process often running its course in less than a day, cholera took on the moniker of "the blue death," as the victim's capillaries ruptured and tinged the skin. Interfering with the small intestine, the blood typically turned "thick and tar-like,"[21] and the heart rate grew increasingly irregular. Dehydrated limbs shriveled before the physician's eyes, but the nervous system remained intact until the end. The victim was, as a rule, fully conscious and in pain until the end of their life.

John Snow, who was born into a relatively impoverished family, could cite his origins when it came to his approach to cholera. William Snow, John's father, was a coal laborer in York, situated to the north toward the Scottish border. The only advantage to the young Snow's childhood location was York's history as the most preeminent city in England in former times. His proximity to Scotland may have served him well, as the northern realm was vibrant with intellectual and medical rigor. Born on March 15, 1813, he was the first of nine children, and soon after his birth, he was baptized by the Reverend G. Brown at All Saints Church, on North Street in Micklegate Ward. The family's headstones can still be recognized in the churchyard.

---

[21] Laura Ball, Cholera and the Pump on Broad Street: The Life and Legacy of John Snow, *The History Teacher*, Vol. 43 no. 1 (Nov., 2009) Society for History Education

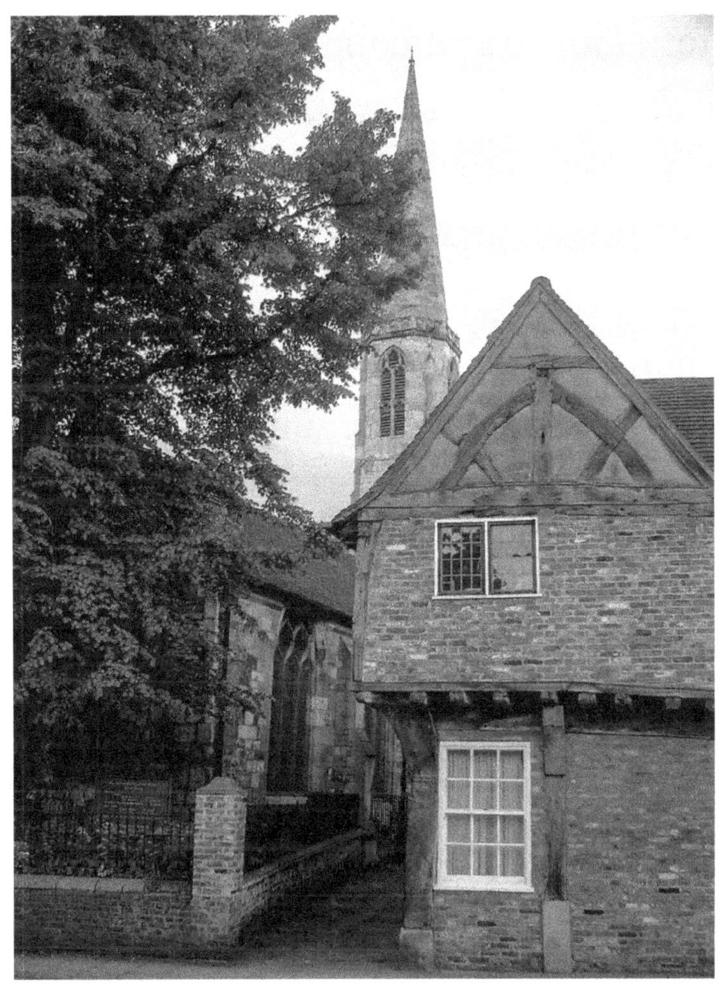

The church where Snow was baptized

York was a walled city from the days of the Roman Empire, and water sources were principally established by wells, less so from rivers. The available water was often contaminated by the market squares, cesspools, ccmctcries and dunghills in the vicinity. For Snow, York was to serve as the appropriate preparation for a youth spent considering the possibility of water-borne disease.

His mother, Frances Snow, was more well-inclined to the benefits of a formal education, and she made note of her son's aptitude for mathematics and science at an early age. She likely shared a gift with her son that was on public display throughout his life, as he continually marked and "thrived on details others overlooked."[22] When the time was right, Frances used a small inheritance in order that her son could attend private school among those of higher economic breeding.

The investment was a sound one as John excelled from the beginning. By the age of 14, he was prepared to serve an apprenticeship to William Hardcastle, the prominent surgeon of Newcastle upon Tyne. He would live and work in that community primarily populated by coal workers from 1827-1833. During that period, he moved from apprentice to serving as Hardcastle's trusted assistant. Little is known of the medical details in Snow's training with Hardcastle, but a fellow apprentice and medical student from Edinburgh, Thomas Giordani Wright, kept a diary. He wrote that the odd appearance of Snow in Newcastle occurred after he was able to "extricate himself from unsatisfactory apprenticeship"[23] near his home.

The time with Hardcastle was apparently a helpful one on two counts. First, his mentor, although hailing from the region, was trained in London and had thus incorporated

---

[22] David Vachon, UCLA Part One, Doctor John Snow Blames Water Pollution for Cholera Epidemic –
www.ph.ucla.edu/epi/snow/fatherofepidemiology.html

[23] Alistair Johnson, John Snow and Thomas Giordani Wright, Medical Apprentices in Newcastle upon Tyne –
www.kora.matrix.msu.edu/files/21/120/15-78-AE-22-snow%20and%20wright%20in%20newcastle-or.pdf

the best available information into his practice. Further, the massive number of coal workers in Newcastle who worked in the surrounding mines presented too heavy a caseload for the available surgeons, and Snow quickly found himself offering medical services with his teacher no longer in the room. The 1831 cholera outbreak in the colliery overwhelmed the town's medical practitioners, and Snow participated in a major outbreak firsthand as a result. The initial impact of it struck a nearby mining village called Killingworth, where the young apprentice grew quickly familiar with the process of the disease. As an "unqualified assistant," he was thrown not only into providing standard treatment above his level of education, but into making grave decisions that were typically entrusted to the senior surgeon.

Snow, like his older colleagues, came to feel the weight of helplessness before the assault, and the most advanced treatments available to him included "disease bleeding laxatives, opium, peppermint and brandy."[24] In his era, much of the available cures were herbal in nature, or alcohol based. The only substance other than normal household items brought to bear on the disease was mercury chloride, which Snow first applied to keelman William Sproat in his lodgings. The patient died within hours. In the following 25 years, tens of thousands died of

---

[24] David Vachon

cholera in England, and these ineffective treatments continued for want of a new alternative. However, the first outbreak inexplicably evaporated as "suddenly and mysteriously"[25] as it had begun by the second year. The loss of life was nearly 50,000 across Britain.

Snow's medical studies under Hardcastle came to a close at the age of 18 as his general interest in disease expanded. The frustration of certain ailments that eluded him drove his already formulating views on the possibility of water being the source of cholera. Most of the miners he had treated spent their time predominantly underground, and Snow theorized that cholera was spread by invisible germs on the hands as the coal laborers had no water for washing.

By the age of 20, Snow had relocated to nearby Burnopfield for a subsequent apprenticeship. However, he returned frequently to Newcastle, a distance of only 10 miles, for a new series of lectures at Bell's Hall initiated by a small group of medical practitioners. For a fee of two guineas, equivalent to approximately $500 today, he took advantage of courses in chemistry, surgery, anatomy, and physiology. If he attended all the courses, Snow was probably on a scholarship from either his uncle, Charles Empson, or family friend Robert Stephenson. Empson was a successful seller of rare art books, while Stephenson

[25] David Vachon

was invested in high-speed locomotives.

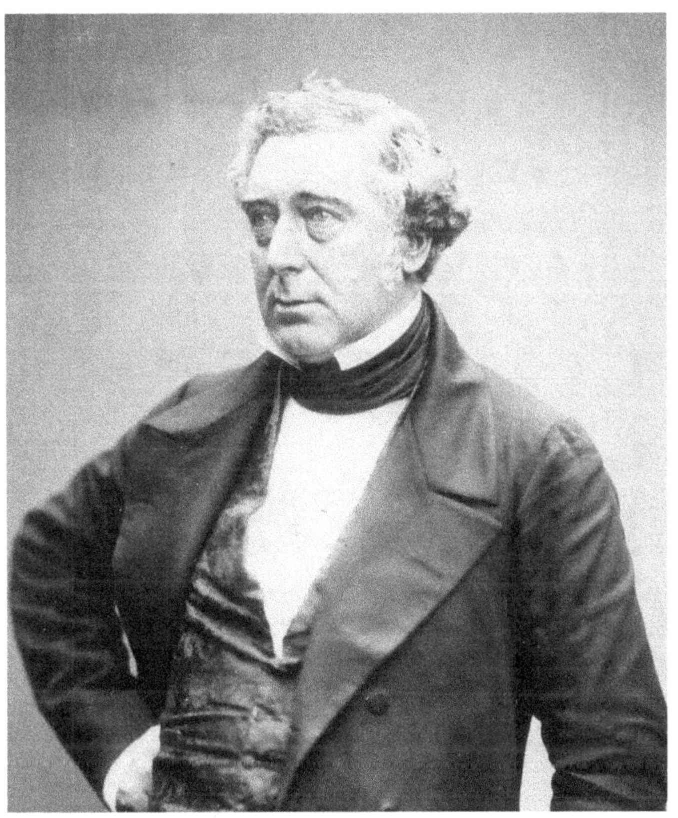

Stephenson

In 1833, Snow began a new assistantship under a Dr. Warburton at Pateley Bridge in Yorkshire. Although little is known of Warburton, Snow wrote admiringly of his mentor over an 18-month period, and being closer to home might have been a comforting experience had he not previously angered residents for his past work in establishing temperance societies there. A standard component of a medical apprenticeship held that the student must neither drink, gamble, nor marry, and Snow held on to those principles throughout his life other than drinking an occasional glass of wine in later years.

The Outbreak in London

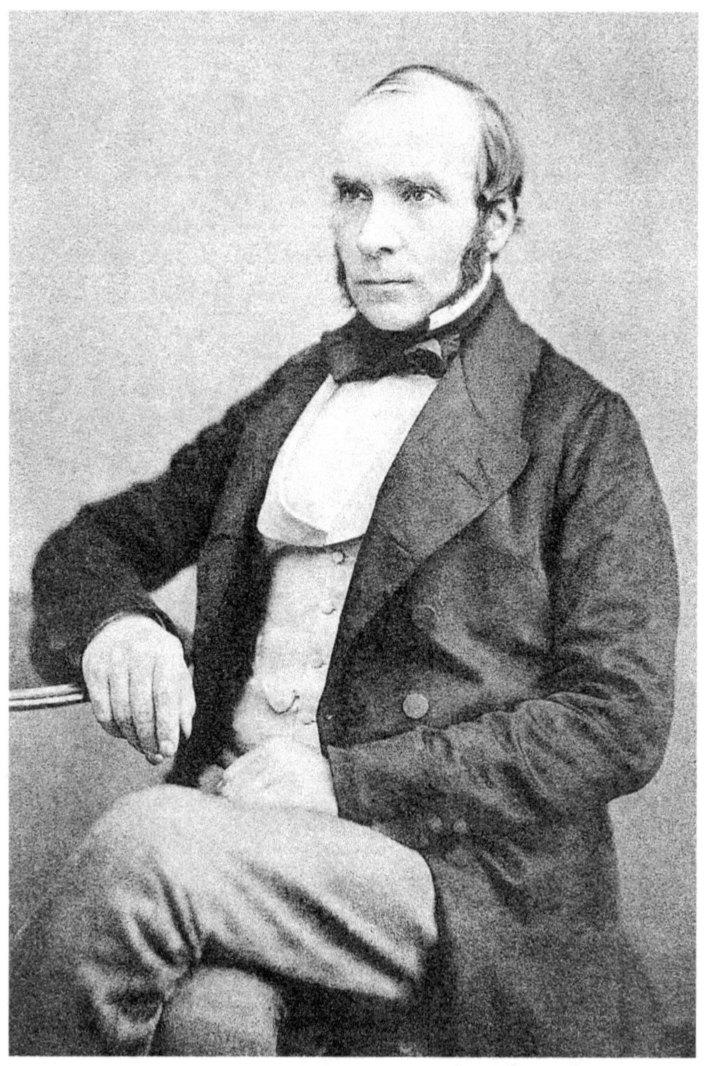

Snow as an adult

Following his term with Warburton, Snow left the region at last for London, covering the entire distance of 400 miles on foot. Once he arrived, he became a student at the Hunterian School of Medicine on Great Windmill Street. In the year that he first witnessed city life in London, 21 medical schools had been established, and Hunterian was likely his first choice due to its comparatively low cost.

Located in the poor Soho district, it was founded in 1769 by Scottish pioneers in medicine and surgery.

In order to be licensed as a surgeon and apothecary, requirements set by the Royal College of Surgeons and the Society of Apothecaries had to be successfully completed. Courses were held daily over a six-month period with an emphasis on chemistry and medical jurisprudence, followed by three months of surgical demonstrations, botany, and general medicine. The cost was roughly equivalent to $7,000 today, a bargain considering the astronomical expenses of modern medical schools.

After two years of this regimen, Snow was accepted as a member of the Royal College. The Hunterian experience and time spent at the Westminster Medical School was in hindsight an ideal opportunity for dissecting the human body. Such access to cadavers were essential in preparations for the Royal Medical and Chirurgical Society. An unfamiliar term to modern society, "chirurgical" is simply an alternative word for surgery as a procedure.

Upon the date of his acceptance, Snow was free to establish a private practice, which he eventually did at nearby 54 Firth Street. From this location, he was able to maintain regular attendance at the outpatient clinic of

Charing Cross Hospital, associated with Westminster. In 1837, he began a term of service at the Westminster Hospital of London before gaining full membership in the Royal College of Physicians the following year. This prestigious body had received its royal charter three centuries prior. Led by humanist and priest Thomas Linacre, King Henry VIII affirmed its status as a college soon after.

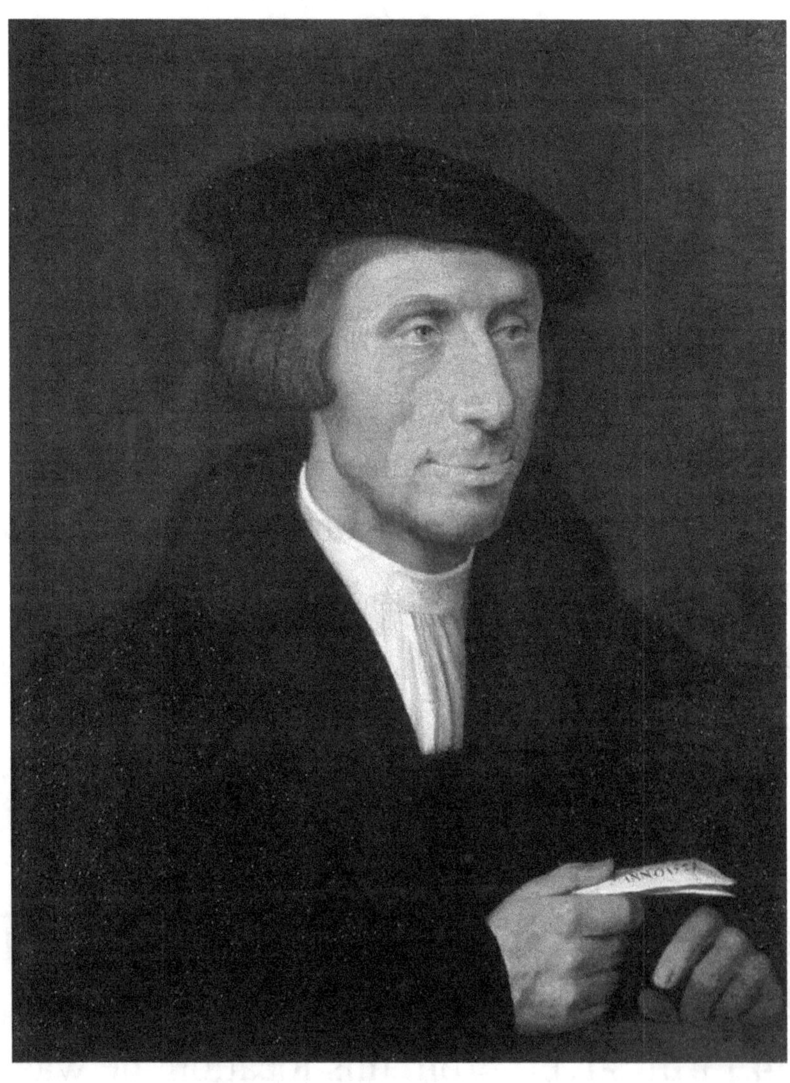

Linacre

Four years later, on October 14, 1841, Snow raised the courage to present his first paper to the London medical community, entitled *On Asphyxia, and on the Resuscitation of Stillborn Children.* With an introductory section of an already well-observed and familiar phenomenon, he proceeded to advocate a cold environment for the stillborn, observing that mammals die far more slowly at temperatures well below that of the body and blood. This suggestion ran counter to some medical views of the day. At the time, stillborn children represented one out of 20 newborn babies. Snow further advocated for a mouth-to-mouth procedure above the use of bellows, which he claimed could not duplicate natural respiration. He ventured into more intricate territory by offering thoughts on various gaseous mixtures of oxygen with standard atmosphere, made the case for occasional use of electric shock, and discussed the physiology of the brain's quest for triggering the initiation of respiration. Although generally disapproving of mechanical technology when natural processes were readily available, Snow developed significant improvements to the anesthetic inhaler. In his preference toward natural resuscitation, he included oral initiation, increased assistance to the chest, and a technique referred to as "Marshall Hall's." Named for a contemporary physiologist who made early breakthroughs in saving drowning victims, the procedure resembles the modern

"Schäfer method." The victim is turned face down, and intermittent pressure is applied to the thorax at a rate of 15 actions per minute.

Snow's paper was published one month after the lecture in the *London Medical Gazette*. Of note is that his live presentation ended with a demonstration of a Mr. Read's "double air pump," somewhat akin to a primitive ventilator. This was ironic, as Snow had just openly discouraged such technologies in favor of more tactile treatment.

In the course of obtaining full credentials as an M.D., Snow graduated from the medical school of the University of London in 1844, at which time he could at last catch sight of employing the term "Doctor." For the esteemed designation, studies in French and Latin added to classes in philosophy and logic. In the British medical structure, practitioners of internal medicine carried the title, where those treating external conditions were knowns as barbers or barber-surgeons.

Snow would not present another paper until 1847, his first as a fully recognized physician and surgeon. This one dealt with the latest updates on anesthetic techniques, entitled *On the Inhalation of the Vapor of Ether*. He had by this point in his career anesthetized a total of 77 patients, which at the time was nearly nonexistent across the empire and had been emphatically resisted where it was employed. The extensive study of gases required to initiate such treatments was an ideal body of knowledge for addressing his continuing fascination with the transmission of cholera and other diseases. He had worked on a scientific presentation on the use of arsenic for the preservation of bodies, but he was forced to abandon it as the toxic effects were causing the attending medical students to fall ill.

Snow spent much of 1848 writing a small pamphlet entitled *On the Mode of Communication of Cholera,* to be published the following year. It was said in his time that Snow understood the mechanisms of "vaporizing volatile"[26] anesthetic agents more deeply than any of his contemporaries. Even heads of the Royal Medical and Chirurgical Society declared that the young physician was "more extensively conversant with its operation, and more successful in administering it, than any living person."[27] Part of the resistance to the fledgling science was due to the brutal nature of the agent's administration, which was devoid of any semblance of finesse, whether by ether or chloroform. Religious denominations had a penchant for viewing any medical technology as a usurpation of God's will, which governed the medical destiny of all humans.

---

[26] Michael A.E. Ramsay, John Snow, MD: Anaesthetist to the Queen of England and Pioneer Epidemiologist, Baylor University Medical Center, January 2006, - www.nchi.nih.gov/pmc/articvles/PMC1352279

[27] Laura Ball

However, Snow's tenacity resulted in safer chemicals and more finely calibrated dosages, vastly preferable to soaked handkerchiefs spread over the face. Lauded as possessing a mastery over the "mechanics" of anesthetics only enhanced his reputation, since to the non-medical citizen, dealing with gases had no apparent "mechanisms." To those unfamiliar with the science, the new treatment was entangled with some form of wizardry, and no doubt based on the fact that it seemed to take a person to the edge of death in order to spare them the pain of full consciousness. To Snow's contemporaries, it must have appeared like an intrusion of the contract between man and God. Science had failed thus far to prove itself in the epidemic crises, and religion was seemingly all that remained for many.

Of course, the paper on the spread of cholera was not written merely out of unprovoked intellectual curiosity. History has categorized outbreaks of the disease with various terms and durations, but regardless of artificial timelines, it raged throughout much of the world for years on end, and what is referred to as the Third Pandemic was not an overstatement. Fatalities ran high in Africa, Asia, and North America as well. This was added to the one million lives lost in Russia, all over a 30-year period that commenced a decade before Snow's paper.

His response to the British outbreak, during which the

nation lost 23,000, began with the tracking of its first victim. John Harnold had visited by boat from Hamburg, going ashore to rent a room in the London community of Horsleydown. There, he died within hours of arrival. Snow spoke to his physician, who was treating a second man named Bleckinsop in the same room a few days after. His subsequent death indicated the presence of a contagion. Suspicion held that the room had not been cleaned between the two guests. Knowing that such deaths always began with gastrointestinal discomfort, the source was narrowed down to either polluted water or food.

  As one of many practitioners in the city of London dealing with cholera, Snow's ability to penetrate prevailing medical traditions was scant. However, by 1853, his growing reputation among the leading early anesthesiologists increased both his confidence and access to public input. In an unexpected and advantageous association with the royal family, he met privately with Prince Albert, Victoria's consort. According to Baylor University Medical Center's Michael A.E. Ramsay, Snow entered the meeting as "the most accomplished anesthetist in the British Isles."[28] Friend and biographer Sir Benjamin Richardson documented the royal encounter with Albert, observing that Snow "returned much pleased"[29] with his reception. He added that Snow was surprised and

---

[28] Chloe Foussianes, Victoria, the True Story of John Snow's Cholera Breakthrough, *Town and Country Magazine*, Feb. 4, 2019

[29] Chloe Foussianes

delighted by Albert's natural kindness, and the royal's intelligent grasp of so many scientific points in the conversation.

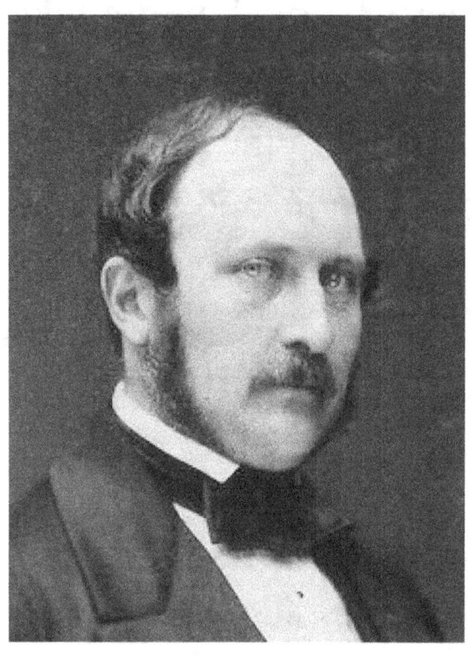

Albert

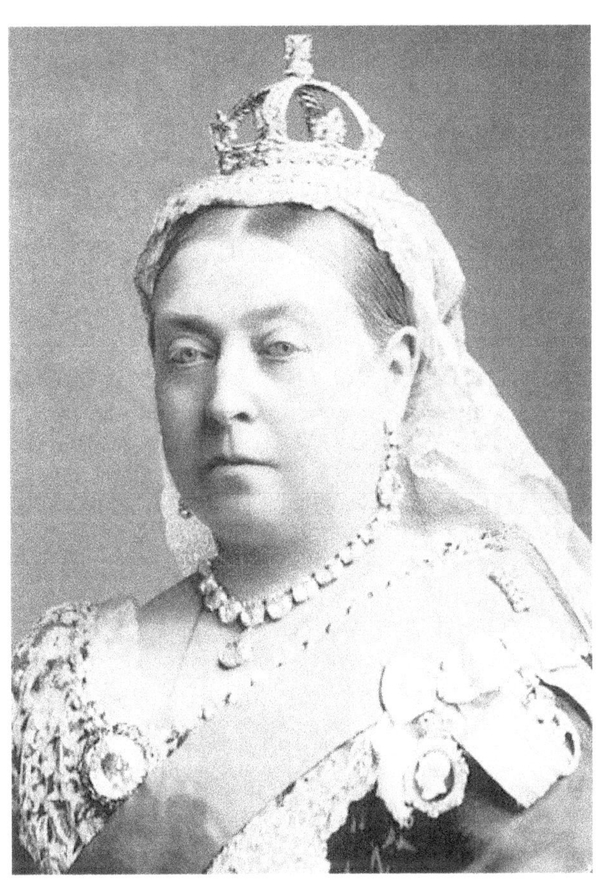

Victoria

The culmination of Albert's inquiry resulted in a summons to the palace to assist Queen Victoria during the birth of Prince Leopold. During his time with the queen, Snow administered an anesthetic, drawing unparalleled ire from medical publications such as *The Lancet*. However, once the news of Victoria's treatment reached the ears of the public, Snow was cast in the unfamiliar role of a national celebrity. An incessant line of curious citizens stopped him on the street with mundane questions regarding the monarch, and of his mysterious practice. Anesthetics, always a delicate procedure, are now common throughout the world, but in a 19th century nation in which the practice was unknown, the public experienced visions of enchanted spells cast over their beloved monarch. As the new medical sensation, Snow clung tenaciously to doctor-client privilege when beset with "royal" questions, and he responded repeatedly with the remark that "Her Majesty is a model patient."[30] He added in private moments that this catch-phrase was absolutely true, and that Victoria's courage in undergoing an unfamiliar medical art with such calm was indeed extraordinary.

Whether Albert or Victoria herself consulted with Snow on the cholera outbreak is unknown, but either way, as Snow entered the cholera debates at the highest level, it was his unchallenged supremacy as an anesthetist that gained him admittance, backed by the highest recommendation in the land. Although this was more than helpful in gaining the right to speak for the water-borne theory of cholera transmission, he was not innately trusted in the field. To make matters worse, he was not an ideal ambassador in either appearance or rhetorical suave, adding to his already poor showing. Rumor held that Snow suffered from a serious speech impediment, but his good friend Richardson never made references to a stutter or other dysfunction in his notes. He did readily concede

------

[30] Chloe Foussianes

that his companion was "modest and rather backward,"[31] and that he was a "poor speaker with a husky voice."[32]

Snow's nearly anonymous document on cholera transmission had been buried among thousands of medical commentaries written during the decade, many of which were authored by prestigious practitioners and sold by prominent publishing houses. Conversely, Snow's was self-published at a cost of many times his monthly income, and only his newfound fame with the royal family elevated the document into upper-tier discussions. The debate had been touched off in 1849 when Snow appeared to speak at the Westminster Medical Society. Perhaps owing to his fame in other specialties, chief critic Dr. James Bird conceded a small show of deference, admitting a possible person-to-person contagion, but utterly downplayed the possibility of water acting as an agent. He gave no credence whatsoever to Snow's description of a tangible "poison" related to the affliction as none had yet been proven to exist. According to the general rules of evidence, Snow was still in a weak position – though he was certain of his theory due to his vast experience with the disease, he had produced no clinical proof of cholera's inner dynamics.

In 1854, the next phase of the earlier outbreak hit the

[31] Ralph M. Waters, John Snow, First Anesthetist, *Bios* Vol. 17 No. 1 (March, 1936) Beta Beta Beta Biological Society

[32] Ralph M. Waters

district of Soho near the very location of Snow's medical practice. In the space of just a few weeks, 700 were killed by the virus in the localized assault. The deadliest of the waves of disease to reach Britain to this point, the epidemic is thought to have erupted in India, and more specifically Bengal.[33] From there, it spread to Russia, then Europe and the U.S. Exacerbating the spread was the presence of 10,000 British troops stationed in India at the time.

The epidemic struck in largely the same geographical pattern as it had two decades earlier, and it caught Britain in the "same state of unpreparedness."[34] The Central Board of Health had been dissolved after the previous outbreak on the assumption that the disease was successfully banished from Britain. Government organizations fell into the trap of believing that one or a few initial cases were not a danger to the country, and that containment was possible. Still unable to provide evidence that could be witnessed through the lens of a microscope, the arrival of cholera at Snow's doorstep opened vast possibilities for identifying its specific medium through statistical means.

By this point in the mutually impotent argument, the single case of Asiatic cholera that led to a death in

---

[33] Britannica.com, Cholera Through History – www.britannica.com/science/cholera/cholera-through-history/

[34] History Home.UK, A Web of English History, Cholera Comes to Britain: October 1831 – www.historyhome.comk.uk/peel/p-health/cholera3.htm

Greenwich was one year gone, making containment unlikely. Following that, three cases were reported on a Prussian vessel in Hull with 10 crewmen on board, but the debate raged on with little evidence to support either side. A month after that, three cases had been reported on a convict ship opposite the Royal Arsenal at Woolwich. The government's obligatory explanation was finally tested on the public and proved extraordinarily weak. As had so many civilizations had in the past, authorities fell back on the idea that the immorality of the poor was responsible for the carnage, and that only those who had "debauched"[35] were dying. The financial network burdened with the task of sustaining Britain's national prosperity considered the poor as a drag on the larger prosperity, and therefore the elite were relatively unconcerned. Moralizing disease evoked the usual debate between the importance of the economy versus the lives in danger of being lost. Large business interests seemed to reach a consensus that a mortality rate of 50% among the lower classes was "acceptable."[36] The first rustlings of the Industrial Revolution also kindled a certain number of profession-related dangers, increasing vulnerability to disease by specific workers.

In the same token, science and the growth of cities harnessed the potential to clean the rivers and upgrade the

[35] The Social Historian, Death in the Time of Cholera – thesocialhistorian.com/death-time-cholera/

[36] Industrialization Diseases

city plumbing, if city leaders would agree to it, but population density made the task all the more difficult. The steam engine could go anywhere, and factories gravitated toward towns and large metropolitan centers. Unemployed rural workers followed, but the result was more waste dumped into the river, and more disease returning through the city pipes. Even the river's entrance into the sea was not immune as cholera could be contracted through shellfish taken from foul water.

The medical profession in Britain faced the daunting pestilence in a state of shock. Armed with little effective knowledge, one physician lamented that cholera was not an innately British phenomenon, and that "other plagues were home-bred."[37] These were too often looked upon with a "fatal indifference"[38] and an assumption of protection based on familiarity. In the decade of the most recent outbreak, international trade trailed off significantly, while the price of food and other items rose, leaving the poor more destitute than ever. All the while, their inability to purchase necessities took a further toll on their general health.

England and most of its colleagues in the "civilized world" were on the cusp of indoor plumbing, which included modern toilets, but these were not available for

---

[37] Laurelyn Douglas, Health and Hygiene in the Nineteenth Century, The Victorian Web, 1991 –
    www.victoriaweb.org/science/health/health10.htm
[38] Laurelyn Douglas

the poorest areas such as Soho. During the first decades of Victoria's reign, baths were rare, and the typical home employed a "privy pail." Water closets were similarly scarce, and towns were often "ankle deep in mud"[39] through entire seasons of the year. Most districts used town wells, fitted with communal pumps for drinking water, soaking, and washing, and septic systems were primitive at best. Most Soho families were in the habit of dumping untreated sewage and animal waste directly into the Thames or into open pits and cesspools underneath the floors of their homes. Where water companies bottled water from the Thames and delivered it directly to pubs, restaurants, breweries and other businesses, private citizens were more bound to the communal pump. It was the age of slaughterhouses and cowsheds in close quarters with bakeries and restaurants, and the characteristics of London hygiene were captured with an eerie accuracy by authors such as Charles Dickens. The supposedly modern city at the heart of the world's greatest empire was experiencing the highest death rate it had seen since the Black Death centuries before. Workers known as "night soil men" were brought in regularly to clear out solid waste from leaky basements, cesspools, or storage tanks outside, and the waste was then sold to farmers as fertilizer. For the middle class and aristocracy, matters were not appreciably better, though the prosperous lived

---

[39] Laurelyn Douglas

in brick houses that absorbed great quantities of moisture.

Soho was one of London's most polluted and densely populated suburbs. According to researcher Susan Bandoni Muench, the district possessed a population density greater than that of modern Manhattan, with the population shut up together in cheap housing with five or six per room. In Soho alone, at least 100,000 lived in a state of poverty, to the point where most scavenged regularly for "rags, bones, coal scraps, and night soil."[40]

In short order, Snow's initial investigation concluded that all the cholera cases of Soho resided within 250 yards of Cambridge Street where it intersected with Broad Street. After 500 cases in a period of 10 days, the map of the occurrences increasingly pointed to a water pump on the Broad intersection. Snow worked around the clock to track down every detail of information available from hospitals and public records. Every avenue was followed to find out who drank from the pump and who did not. Even in the later stages of the outbreak, Snow concluded beyond the shadow of a doubt that "nearly all the deaths had taken place within a short distance of the pump."[41] The success of this line of pursuit went further as hundreds of cases were traced to nearby schools,

[40] Wills, Matthew, John Snow and the Birth of Epidemiology, Daily Jstor.org, May 28, 2018 – www.daily.jstor.org/john-snow-and-the-birth-of-epidemiology/

[41] Sarah Zielinski, Smithsonian Magazine, Cholera, John Snow and the Grand Experiment, August 18, 2010 – www.smithsonianmag.com/science-nature/cholera-john-snow-and-the-grand-experiment-33496891/

restaurants, businesses and pubs. The keeper of one coffee shop was found to have served several glasses of water from the pump leading up to the epidemic and reported that at least nine customers, not all from the area, had come down with the disease. All of these statistics were gathered in a massive sweep of the population conducted by Snow and his assistant, John Joseph Whiting.

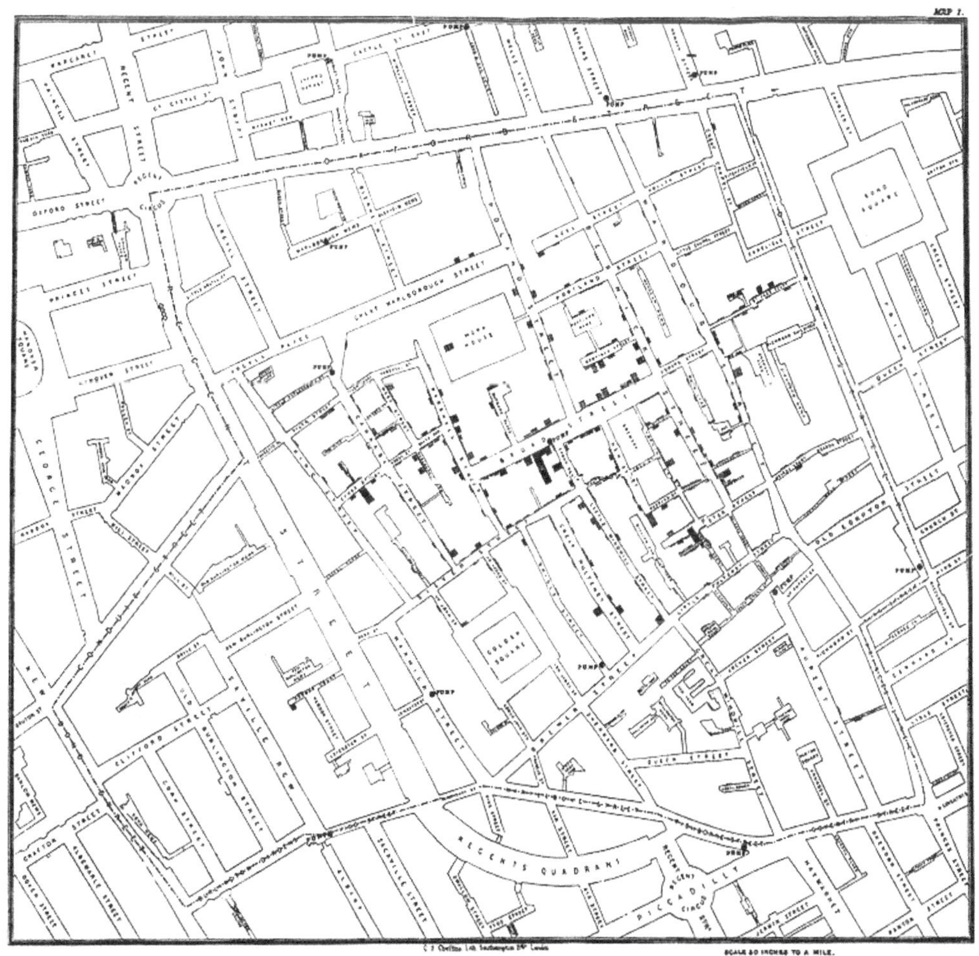

Snow's map of cholera cases

Fortunately, Snow and Whiting lived in an era when the efficiency of city organizations was at its historical best in terms of record-keeping. Britain was always passionately devoted to social statistics, and two decades before the outbreak, the General Register Office of London had begun to keep track of births and deaths within the confines of the city. These records were actually kept for the purpose of transferring wealth by inheritance with greater ease, but Snow was able to use the information for a larger purpose. The Office maintained a system of street addresses with numbers clearly marked on each house, a practice instituted a century earlier. The Register Office established not only who it was that died on any given day or night, but where they died and the cause of death.

Snow made an early visit to the Register Office to collect death certificates for the surrounding population of Golden Square, site of the infamous pump. Armed with the dates, addresses, and data related to the timing of the illness for all the area's victims, he soon established the Broad Street pattern and placed the water pump at the epicenter.

The sudden spate of deaths had already caused a panic in the district, and three-quarters of the population fled within the first six days. Snow subsequently noted, "There is no doubt that the mortality was much diminished, as I said before, by the flight of the population, which commenced soon after the outbreak; but the attacks had so far diminished before the use of the water was stopped, that it is impossible to decide whether the well still contained the cholera poison in an active state, or whether, from some cause, the water had become free from it."

During the first year of the outbreak, Snow and Whiting conducted the world's first study on the differentiated mortality of cholera with water as the source. A second more detailed study was undertaken over the following five years. Visiting the homes of victims became only the first phase of a statistical mission, as the investigation's criteria soon expanded to the two primary water companies serving the city. In addition to manner of death, address, and timing, it was Snow's intention to ascertain from each company the quantity of water available to the families during the period of illness from each company. In addition, he sought to know the periods in which it was to be shut off, and the amounts charged on the water bills. This ushered in a more far-reaching investigation of city-wide proportions.

What was to be called Snow's "Grand Experiment" was a test of the two major water sources serving the city of London. This entailed an effort to support the water-borne theory from the whole of London down to the Broad Street district. Before the 1850s, the Thames had been a relatively clean river, but by mid-century, massive quantities of waste had been dumped directly into its flow. The largest water sources were the Southwark-Vauxhall facility of South London and the Lambeth Waterworks to the north, and the locations of the two companies made such an experiment ideal for a comparative study. Lambeth was established well upriver, and therefore far less likely to be contagious if water was to be proved the answer at all. Indeed, the number of deaths in the areas served by Southwark-Vauxhall reached 375, while Lambeth's area came to 37. Such a finding should have enabled the next step in the chain to prove water contamination. Unfortunately, the direct effect from the two sources on their specific populations was not verified in sufficient detail. The conclusions of the process lacked the force to prevail in either a legal or medical case, and it fell well short of proving either theory in a convincing manner. At the least, a door-to-door canvas would have been required. Even a modern replay of the investigation by a team from the University of British Columbia, with full knowledge that Snow's theory was eventually proven correct, showed that his "Grand Experiment was a failure"[42] in terms of methodology. That said, other studies were not so unkind to Snow's statistics. British physician Arthur Hill Hassall, a contemporary, also investigated the Southwark-Vauxhall and Lambeth Waterworks. In regards to the former, he declared the intake near Battersea Park to be "the most disgusting water I have ever examined.[43]

____

[42] Sarah Zielinski

Nevertheless, the Broad Street fountain remained at the center of the outbreak, and two peripheral oddities drew attention to it as well. Two women, an aunt and her niece, lived a good distance from Soho with no apparent connection to the district's water source. However, when the aunt, Susannah Eley was investigated in an interview with her son, he admitted that she had at one time lived in Soho. He added that she had a soft spot for the water of that particular pump, and it was deemed by others as well to be "colder and more carbonated"[44] than the norm. Related to that, a favorite drink in the area was generally referred to as "sherbet," a mixture of water and a flavored powder that fizzed when mixed in. In this specific area of London, water for such a concoction more often than not came from the Soho pump on Broad Street.

Fond of the "sherbet" concoction, Eley often had bottles of the Broad Street water brought to her as a special treat, and she and her niece each drank it on the day they died. The familiar white flecks floating in their digestive tracts were found. After some work at connecting person-to-person contact and activity around the pump, the disease was ultimately traced back to Sarah Lewis, who had washed the diaper of her son Frances at the pump, a few scant feet from the location of a cesspool.

---

[43] Samantha Hajna, David L. Buckeridge, James A. Hanley

[44] Laura Ball

Pockets of business interests and individual residents who did not come down with the disease were found to have partaken from other water sources. The local workhouse operated its own well, and the others had bought water from Grand Junction Waterworks. Likewise, the local brewery made use of its own well, and no cases were reported among the employees. Among the children, several of the victims had grabbed a quick drink on their walk to school. By all appearances, the contents of the washed diaper had been thrown into the cesspool and leaked into the drinking water source.

More certain than ever of his theory, Snow again undertook the arduous task of convincing the powerful and pedigree members of the medical brotherhoods of London. The London medicial experts regularly discussed such matters at length from their more protected estates. Not only did Snow lack pedigree, but he was socially ill-at-ease as well, overly shy and not a fluent speaker. However, whenever he entered the halls of advanced medical learning, he continued to carry the advantage of being the acknowledged master of anesthesiology throughout the land, and such a status continued to sustain his right to speak, as well as the medical community's obligation to listen. Furthermore, the association with the Royal Family still lent an air of validity to his right to seek a majority of advocates for his position.

In the early phase of his investigation, Snow's evidence for the water theory was largely circumstantial, but he knew a great deal about the lives of his neighbors only a few streets away from his residence, issues that could not be taught in medical school. According to one biographer, Snow was not just a "health tourist goggling at all the pain and death."[45] Originating in a family environment in much the same condition as his London neighbors, Snow refused to blame the disease on the habits of the poor, and he objected vociferously when they were maligned. He insisted, "The poor were dying in disproportionate numbers not because they suffered from moral failings – they were being poisoned."[46]

The battle lines were clearly drawn for the debate. Snow's *On the Mode of Communication of Cholera* proposed that a not-yet-understood "cholera poison" was not only spread through contaminated food and water, but that it had the capability to multiply itself. Rather than respiratory in nature, cholera was, according to Snow's determined insistence, digestive in nature, a "local affliction of the bowels"[47] caused by an intake of *materies morbi*. These agents of contagion were characterized as disease-producing particles from fecal material found in drinking water.

[45] Dierdre Mask, How the Father of Epidemiology Made the Connection Between Disease and Geography, Time, April 14, 2020 – www.time.com/5820194/addresses-epidemiology/

[46] Dierdre Mask

[47] Sick City Project

Although the document eventually became known to the medical community, it was met with general apathy and with utter silence from the general population, few of whom were even aware of it. Until the pamphlet's second incarnation some years later, as well as 20th century reprints decades after the epidemic, Snow's brief treatise on cholera sold a grand total of 56 copies out of 100 that were printed.

On the other side of the argument stood the miasma theory, the British descendant of the ancient Greek system of "humours." The powerful Royal College of Surgeons stood by the airborne theory from the revelation of the first case. Several had experienced it in India years before, which further hardened the resolve of their argument and dismissed any suggestion of inexperience. In agreement with the idea that the disease originated in rotting matter, the miasma theory held that it was a poisonous form of bad air emitted from decaying organic material that sickened the citizens. Germs held no sway with the origination of disease in the 1850s, and few physicians believed that the two were even connected.

The dismissal of the germ theory extended to numerous other diseases as well. The "miasma" view was supported by leading figures of medical organizations, including Edwin Chadwick and the legendary Florence Nightingale, who became pivotal in the entrance of women into the nursing profession. Ironically, both could point to the natural dangers of Soho to prove their point. As one of London's "liveliest and filthiest districts,"[48] it was easy to accept that either the air or the water was of sufficiently lower quality, and that the air could thus have been the cause of the outbreak. The proposed gases of the miasma theory were supposed to jump the barrier to various other sites in the body, but such an idea was unworkable to Snow, who according to contemporaries "really knew his gasses"[49] as an anesthesiologist. In fact, unbeknownst to the medical community, he regularly experimented on himself with new varieties of experimental "vapors."

With the idea of polluted vapors jumping systemic barriers, support of the miasma idea was not so illogical, and it was only reinforced by the foul olfactory conditions of London in later years, known as the "Great Stink." In deference to the Greek theories, the Black Death and chlamydia were spread by air pollution, commonly referred to as "night air." These conditions supported an airborne hypothesis with enough strength to refute Snow's unproven germ theory.

Despite the fierce debate, those of the miasma school were more driven by despair and want of a proven alternative theory, not by bold analysis. Added to

---

[48] Sick City Project

[49] David Vachon

London's woes was a suspicion on the part of the "miasmists" that the bone-boiling factories were in part to blame. Plants that dissolved animal tissue resulted in products such as soap and glue, and the miasma proponents found in the bone-boiling institution a perfect model for their theory of polluted air. Snow, always skeptical that foul air would transfer to the intestinal tract so easily, immediately pointed out that the bone-boiling workers were not dying of cholera. The effect of factory odors to the workforce was generally of a low exposure, but proponents of the airborne theory were invested in the accumulation of long-term effects, despite the fact that cholera normally moved with such rapidity.

Regardless of the affiliation to one or other of these theories, neither camp was able to prove beyond any doubt that theirs was the correct one. Majority opinion, pedigree, and the economy were brought to bear by the traditional advocates, not scientific proof. As in the present day, several of the "well-funded industries"[50] had a prodigious financial stake in the outcome of such inquiries, including the bone-boiling factories. While waiting, the politically superior traditionalists maintained supremacy despite enjoying no certainty of anything.

In the face of Snow's yet incomplete case, the entire human response to cholera was surrender. Lamentably,

---

[50] Dale P. Sandler

with the traditional belief in the miasma theory, even more waste was dumped into the Thames, increasing the danger. Cholera would not be "banished for good"[51] until well after the outbreak subsided, following the "Great Stink" when the overburdened river reached its tipping point. Worse, diseases such as smallpox and typhoid did not wait their turn, taking advantage of the population's weakened condition to erupt in similar fashion. All the major health dangers, typhoid in particular, became associated with the sea as international travel heightened the problem, and London's failure to "recognize and isolate"[52] the new emergence of cholera allowed greater carnage than ever before. Mitigation proceeded blindly, and the distance covered by the disease was far too vast for containment.

One opponent, John Simon, dubbed Snow as "peculiar,"[53] a weighty term in coded British speech. A difficult rival to thwart, Simon was a pathologist, surgeon, and public health officer who would go on to become the first Chief Medical Officer to Victoria's government, and later the President of the Pathological Society of London. His numerous essays on public health problems in the city of London were well-respected. Simon took issue with Snow's theory, writing, "This doctrine is, that cholera

---

[51] Science Museum, Brought to Life, Cholera Comes to Victorian London –
www.broughttoilife.sciencemuseum.org.uk/broughttolife/themes/publichealth/cholera

[52] Industrialization Diseases, Cholera and Great Britain – www.industrializationdiseases.wordpress.com/cholera-and-great-britain/

[53] Smithsonian Magazine

propagates itself by a 'morbid matter' which, passing from one patient in his evacuations, is accidentally swallowed by other persons as a pollution of food or water; that an increase of the swallowed germ of the disease takes place in the interior of the stomach and bowels, giving rise to the essential actions of cholera, as at first a local derangement; and that 'the morbid matter of cholera having the property of reproducing its own kind must necessarily have some sort of structure, most likely that of a cell."

Moreover, Simon called into question several of what were considered Snow's quirky habits at the time. One was an adherence to temperance, and another his completely vegetarian diet. He raised Snow's status as an ongoing bachelor and expressed skepticism that his colleague had ever entertained a romance of any sort. In a prestigious medical world inhabited by men of pedigree, Snow, by contrast, dressed like a commoner and was never seen with friends. In concert with *The Lancet's* Chief Editor Thomas Wakley, constant pressure was exerted on the once rural physician and his minority theory by means of personal attack and innuendo.

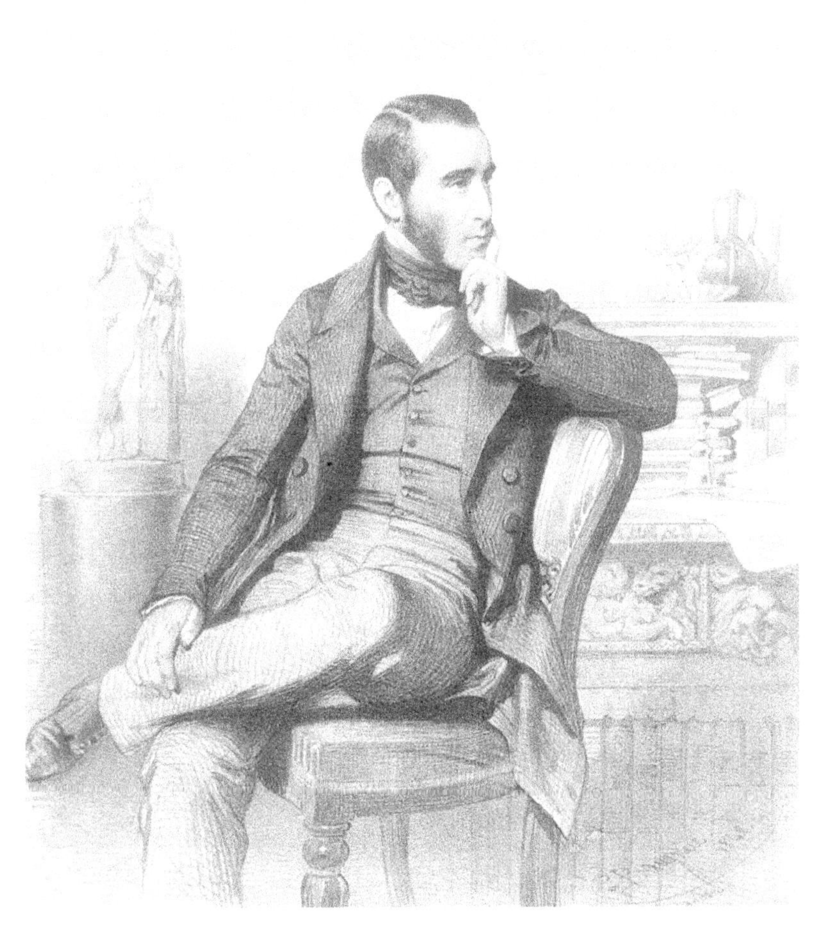

A lithograph of Simon

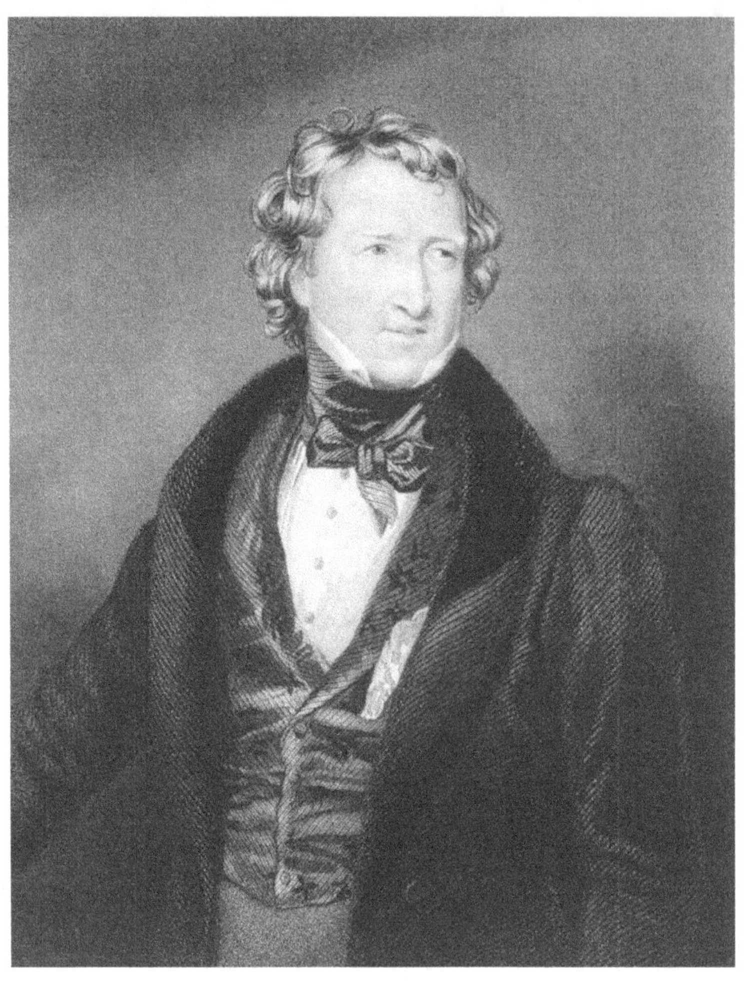

Wakley

Once Snow's theory was proven correct, opposing forces still refused to give in, pretending they had never heard of the affirming research. In the same vein, foreign medical associations maintained their professional nationalism by ignoring his achievement as the ramblings of a commoner. A competition extended to the world by the French with an award of 1,200 pounds for the discovery of a process that would control cholera ignored Snow's findings altogether.

A few opponents were, to the contrary, successfully won over. Among them was the Reverend Henry Whitehead, a local priest who took it upon himself to prove Snow wrong. Whitehead interviewed a woman living at 40 Broad Street who had contracted cholera from another source. Enough such cases, he believed, would be sufficient to sink Snow's belief that the pump was to blame for "the most terrible attack of cholera which ever occurred in this kingdom."[54] Unable to find the body of evidence for which he had hoped, Whitehead moved away from those officials who contended that sewage could not have leaked from town pipes into the pump. Abandoning the miasma theory, his conclusion was the same as Snow's: the diaper in question, once cast off, leaked from the cesspool and mingled with the pump water.

[54] Kathleen Tuthill

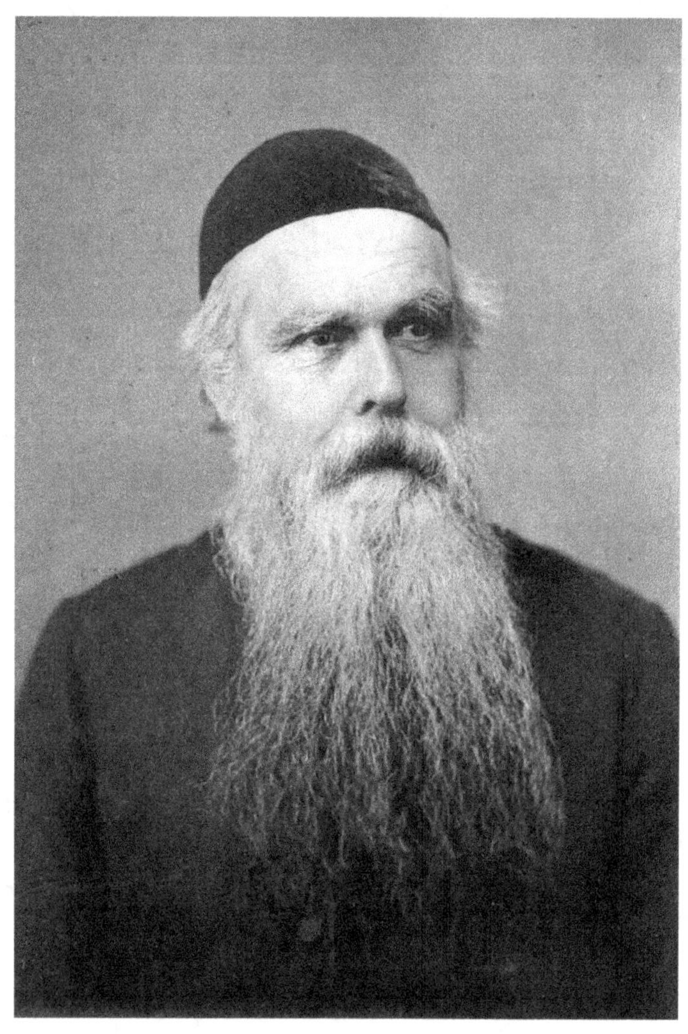

Whitehead

Even with corroborating evidence from the locale, Snow's visibility in the conflict did not improve. The *Mode of Communication of Cholera*, written by an obscure practitioner in a poor part of the city, could not rise to the top. Snow had never held a public health office or a university position. Despite his groundbreaking work with anesthesia, he was widely characterized as a "crank"[55] who poked holes in the works and theories of his

[55] Sick City Project

professional betters. Along with rejection of the germ theory came a deaf ear for his plea to "provide ample supply of water free from contamination"[56] and "effect good and proper drainage."[57]

Throughout the Soho outbreak, the recalcitrant Thomas Wakley lamented having no alternative to Snow's theory, which he despised. Wakley, against all logic, continued to trumpet the status quo in *The Lancet*, though he also conceded he lacked faith in his own position: "All is darkness and confusion, vague theory and a vain speculation."[58] He added that in his present day, there were more questions than workable theories, and more surrender than conclusive analysis. Clearly, the miasma supporters could not identify the disease other than through related scourges, as Wakley noted: "Is it a fungus, an insect, a miasma, an electrical disturbance, a deficiency of ozone, a morbid off-scouring from the intestinal canal?"[59] Ultimately, Wakley threw up his hands and concluded, "We know nothing, we are at sea in a whirlpool of conjecture."[60]

The miasma theory appealed to both sanitary reformers in London, and to the medical movement toward

---

[56] Sick City Project

[57] Sick City Project

[58] Ph.ucla.edu, Cholera; Brief History During the Snow Era (1813-1858) – www.ph.ucla.edu/snow/1859map/cholera_prevailingtheories_a.2.html

[59] Ph.ucla.edu

[60] Ph.ucla.edu

environmental hygiene over personal health, which neatly explained disease among the poor. A second theory entered the ring as well with nearly the same level of resistance as there was to Snow: the "blood generation theory." This theory argued that there was a "spontaneous generation of disease in the blood."[61] No source was attributed to such a "generation," which is little surprise since it defied the medical logic of the era. Predominantly a German proposal, it gained little support among British practitioners. In the end, such neglect delayed acceptance of Snow's germ theory.

Equally ignored, even in his home country of Italy, was the work of Filippo Pacini, whose career paralleled Snow in many ways. He discovered and analyzed the actual cholera organism by microscope in 1854. In a laboratory to the northwest of Florence, his discovery of the "comma-shaped" bacillus was to bear the name *of Vibrio cholerae Pacini.* The tangible proof for which Snow had labored in pursuit of an active organism, Pacini's *contagium vivum* was entirely ignored across Europe and Britain. Had international borders not been so zealously defended by academics, a unified proposal could have been put forward by the Snow and Pacini schools of thought.

---

[61] Ph.ucla.edu

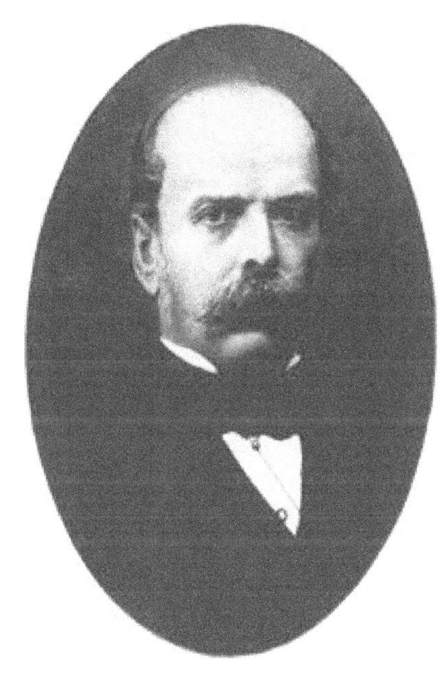

Pacini

In the most intense year of the outbreak, Snow had rivals who served as collegial advocates of similar theories to his. Where they disagreed was in the hunt for final credit, and each accused the other of prizing the public rewards for discoveries over care for the loss of human life. Chief among them was William Budd, a British physician who had trained in Paris and at the University of Edinburgh. Working in Bristol, Budd was known for tracing a typhoid epidemic to a group of revelers, of which eight died following a gathering after ingesting tainted lemonade. Only one month after the publication of Snow's *Mode of Communication of Cholera*, Budd published *Malignant Cholera: Its Propagation and Its Prevention*. In terms of the debate over whether water or air was the source of cholera, Snow beat Budd to at least a statistical victory for his hypothesis by 10 days. Where Snow was granted a densely packed workshop for his study, Budd's case was based on thorough surveys of rural outbreaks. In the long term, he erred by proposing a fungal basis to his theory, while conceding the possibility of water and air as possible culprits.

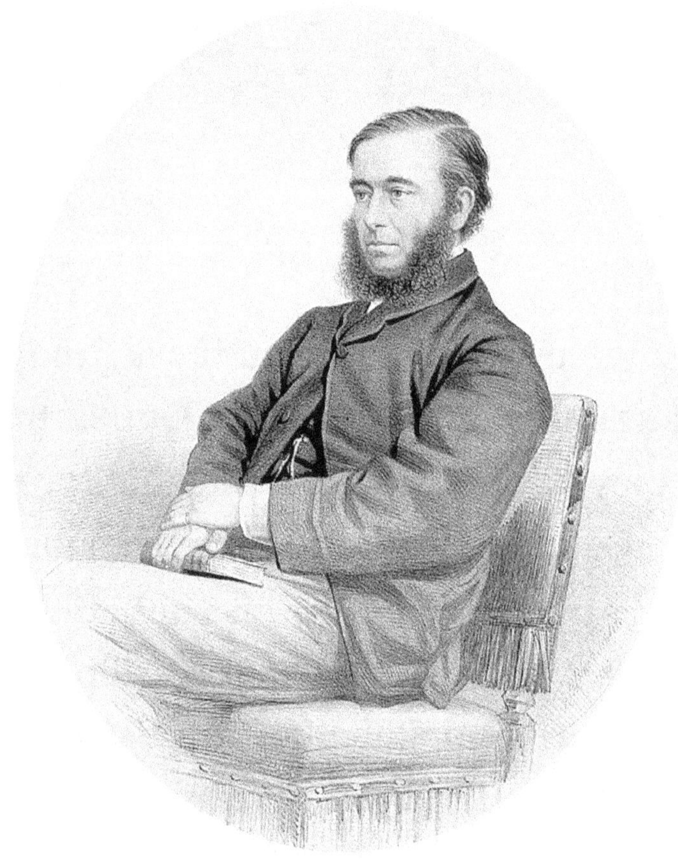

Budd

Snow gradually honed his findings to eliminate air. He had studied so much related matter to the microbic and fungal theories in vogue at the time that he felt confident in making a final declaration. He was certain that the contagious agent was one that attacks the intestinal mucosa without passing into the blood stream, and he deemed the nose, lungs, and blood as irrelevant in terms of the disease's pathway. Like Pacini, Snow concluded that without a doubt, the entity that promulgated cholera was able to "multiply itself…changing surrounding materials to its own nature."[62] Budd went in an almost identical direction, making note of the Bristol Medico-Chirurgical Society's discovery of "peculiar microscopic objects,"[63] entirely in keeping with the "rice-water" discharges described by ancient physicians, only under magnification. Finally, he adopted the idea of an active, multiplying virus, but he continued to include air as another vehicle for the illness' distribution.

The opposition continued to reject anything that resembled an organism that appeared to possess life. The white flecked particles were "not fungi, but food taken,"[64] evidenced by residual particles of meals. "Fungi" was the nearest the establishment would come to involving the "germ," but they were not the same. The German physician Liebig took Snow's certainties even further by embracing the concept of molecular changes brought about by the agent, preferable to "vague notions on animalcules and fungi."[65]

[62] P.E. Brown, John Snow, the Autumn Loiterer, *Bulletin of the History of Medicine*, Vol. 35 No. 6, (Nov., -Dec., 1961) Johns Hopkins University Press

[63] P.E. Brown

[64] P.E. Brown

[65] P.E. Brown

Realizing that Snow had won the race in the eyes of the medical community and the public, Budd made an artful maneuver in their cantankerous relationship. He conceded the bragging rights of first publication to his adversary while refusing to admit that the two theories were even similar, all in an effort to attain independent success when his was eventually chosen. Budd swore that his conclusions owed nothing at all to Snow or his work, and while he would let Snow have the credit for the first discovery, he was clear that his own work would be judged more highly on the "intrinsic superiority"[66] of a more advanced and honed theory.

In the end, Budd may have been correct, as Snow became primarily known for the social tracing of the disease to its correct source and its vehicle. He identified the "poison" as an organism capable of multiplying, but not the specific ingredients and clinical mechanics of cholera's ability to overwhelm the interdependent network of human systems. Nonetheless, Budd lost much of his place in history by coming to print and the podium nearly two weeks late. Only a few months later, Snow became President of the London Medical Society, from which he became an early proponent of clinically relevant research. In hindsight, modern scholars consider Snow to be the practitioner who connected the "three realms of bedside,

---

[66] P.E. Brown

hospital, and laboratory medicine."[67]

The appointment would not come until after Snow's victory in Broad Street was made complete. Amid two alternate studies of the Broad Street breakout, one local and another undertaken by England's General Board of Health, he was the victor in terms of medical and public perception. Delivering his research and arguing his case before Soho town officials on September 7, 1854, Snow convinced them to remove the handle from the pump and render it non-functional. The local officeholders were still reluctant to believe him, and the miasma theory was hard to kill, but they lived in a "panic-stricken"[68] state of paralysis with no ideas of their own to offer.

Snow explained:

> "On proceeding to the spot, I found that nearly all the deaths had taken place within a short distance of the [Broad Street] pump. There were only ten deaths in houses situated decidedly nearer to another street-pump. In five of these cases the families of the deceased persons informed me that they always sent to the pump in Broad Street, as they preferred the water to that of the pumps which were nearer. In three other

[67] Michael A.E. Ramsay

[68] Scott Crosier, John Snow: The London Cholera Epidemic of 1854 –
www.webprojects.oit.ncsu.edu/project/bio/183de/Black/science/science_reading/8.html

cases, the deceased were children who went to school near the pump in Broad Street ...

"With regard to the deaths occurring in the locality belonging to the pump, there were 61 instances in which I was informed that the deceased persons used to drink the pump-water from Broad Street, either constantly or occasionally ...

"The result of the inquiry then was, that there had been no particular outbreak or prevalence of cholera in this part of London except among the persons who were in the habit of drinking the water of the above-mentioned pump-well.

"I had an interview with the Board of Guardians of St. James's parish, on the evening of Thursday, the 7th September, and represented the above circumstances to them. In consequence of what I said, the handle of the pump was removed on the following day."

To the great surprise of the local officials, the epidemic in Soho trickled to a stop once the pump was shut off. Citizens who had fled the neighborhood early in the outbreak began to return, and the daily regimen stabilized. With Snow's theory about water being the source gaining credence by the hour, public officials who still believed the concept to be nonsense refused to take any further measures. Indeed, despite the apparent success at beating back the disease, they flatly rejected the idea of cleaning up the cesspools and sewers operating beneath their feet. The Board of Health issued its report, and part of it read, "We see no reason to adopt this belief."[69]

One year later, a London magazine called *The Builder* published Snow's complete findings and added a challenge directed at complacent Soho officials. In a stern warning, they were exhorted to repair the sewers at once and close the cesspools and drains. The thematic statement of the piece was to the point: "In spite of late numerous deaths, we have all the materials for a fresh epidemic."[70]

Despite the article's passion and the entirety of Snow's data, it would take many years before Snow's admonition of the dangers of "night soil" were heeded.

Snow's Final Years and Legacy

Snow continued his reign at the summit of modern anesthesia, but his status was not accomplished alone. The idea had persisted since ancient times, but a team in Boston demonstrated the first use of advanced anesthesia, proudly declaring the event "Ether Day."[71] Snow soon

---

[69] Kathleen Tuthill, John Snow and the Broad Street Pump, On the Trail of an Epidemic, UCLA, Department of Epidemiology, Fielding School of Public Health, November, 2003 – www.ph.ucla.edu/epi/snowcricketarticle.html

[70] Kathleen Tuthill

became aware of the American event, having begun working with anesthesia around the same time. To his great displeasure, two Americans, William T.G. Morton and surgeon John Collins Warren, had employed the vapor of diethyl ether with the draped cloth method. In Scotland, Dr. James Y. Simpson had begun administering chloroform for women struggling with pain in childbirth, in much the same manner. A full-time anesthesiologist, Snow had caused a stir among patients by treating the queen, but he repeated the feat seven years later for the birth of Princess Beatrice. Patients who were initially horrified began to browbeat their doctors, explaining that since it was given to the queen, it should be given to them.

For a decade, the idea of an anesthetic for childbirth was severely criticized by the establishment, and it was often considered to be "meddling" in a natural process. The initial failure in accepting the procedure was in large part due to Dr. Simpson's "aggressive style."[72] The treatment consisting of pouring open drops of chloroform onto a fabric inserted over the patient's face was a blunt approach even in that day. Snow, however, was renowned for being "systematic and thorough,"[73] interested in a more gradual process with more safety precautions. In medical presentations, he spoke frequently to the

---

[71] Donald Caton, MD, John Snow's Practice of Obstetric Anesthesia, January 2000, Anesthesiology –
    www.anesthesiology.pubs.asahq.org/article.aspx?aspx=1945835
[72] Donald Caton, MD
[73] Donald Caton, MD

"pathophysiology of adverse reactions."[74] His second book, published in the year of his death, *On Chloroform and Other Anaesthetics: Their Action and Administration*, showed a deft touch and state of enlightenment compared to the comparatively barbaric techniques then at play in both hemispheres. Well into the cholera epidemic, during which Snow treated other ailments as well, the notes taken from 4,000 cases in which he administered anesthetic agents were always with him. The first collection disappeared, and knowledge of his earliest treatments are unknown, but modern scholars are aware that he pursued an exhaustive search for safer vapors than chloroform and diethyl ether. Included among them were chlorated muriatic ether, and what was termed the "Dutch Liquid,"[75] a hydrochlorate of chloride and acetyl. Laudanum is mentioned among his notes for treating postpartum pain, and he carefully calibrated dosages in terms of both quantity and timing. For childbirth, he all but eliminated doses in the first phase, introducing it in the second and thereby taking the patient to "the border of unconsciousness."[76] To improve the function and finesse of mechanical instruments, he devised a new brass vaporizer immersed in water to control the temperature.

In a 12-year period, Snow employed anesthesia in a total

---

[74] Donald Caton, MD

[75] Donald Caton, MD

[76] Donald Caton, MD

of 5,000 procedures. These included dental extractions, lithotomy, lithotripsy, the removal of breast tumors, hemorrhoids, cleft lips, and childbirth, among others. Along the way, he worked in consultation with 32 obstetricians, bringing a delicate hand to the unpredictable process.

John Snow did not live to see the full extent of his theories proven. He died in 1858 at the age of 45 and was interred at the Brompton Cemetery of London. Tragically, though he lived an obsessively healthy life, one professional habit contributed to his early demise. Despite the fact that he "exercised vigorously,"[77] was abstinent, distilled his own water (which was cleaner but with an absence of minerals), and lived a calculated regimen, he had a strong work ethic, and several signs point to unheeded warnings. An early bout with tuberculosis and a proposed Vitamin D deficiency from a regimen of vegetarianism have been cited as potential problems, and while some of these points are open for debate, it was the prolonged habit of experimenting on himself that led to a fatal renal failure typified by swollen fingers. The official cause of Snow's death was a stroke. He never realized that his devotion to the study of anesthetics was so hazardous to his own health, but his self-experimentation was presumably an effort to guard the lives of others from

---

[77] David Vachon

incomplete studies.

  In the years following his death, the Thames River had endured enough, and the years of the "Great Stink" began. In a resounding affirmation of Snow's theory about cholera, it was noted that when the stench reached its peak, the mortality rate did not rise from cholera. However, it also meant that city leaders had not taken to heart the warnings of filth being drawn into the intake of water companies. London was increasingly known to be one of the filthiest cities in the world, a blow to the accustomed superiority of British culture. George Henry Lewes' observation of the era was telling: "Few of us after thirty can claim robust health."[78]

  A persistent myth claims that Snow discovered the cause of cholera, despite his emphatic protestations that he had not. He tracked the source of one outbreak to a successful conclusion and made a plausible investigation of a major city's water source from an increasingly dangerous river. He expertly demonstrated the basis of epidemiological investigation for major outbreaks, a model for what is now used in 21st century medicine. Snow was, once his education permitted, thrown into an era of startling new knowledge and radical uncertainties."[79] He contributed to the new body of knowledge and made excellent use of

---

[78] Laurelyn Douglas

[79] Sick City Project

what had already come to pass. He met the trepidation of his era in impressive historical terms, "courageous and clear-sighted."[80] Through his entire life, he did little else than pursue scientific goals. Even on his deathbed, he was busy penning the final chapter of his work on anesthetics, evidence that his knack for seeing a project through to completion was nearly maniacal. This is ascribed by many to his rural background, which imbued him with a "farm training in responsibility,"[81] partnering with his natural sense of mechanics.

As the outbreaks subsided before the advent of the 20th century, save for one brief episode, Snow's work fell into "general obscurity."[82] However, it was revived by the American activist William Thompson Sedgwick. Despite Snow's level of advancement on bacteriology, he was being outdone by a new generation of scientists armed with greater technology and conceptual discoveries. Still, his lifelong study of the subject was the best example of his own era, and Sedgwick took it seriously. He was a co-founder of the MIT-Harvard School of Public Health, and a prodigious writer. Drawing on Snow's principles, he applied bacteriology to a textbook on "sanitary science."[83]

---

[80] Sick City Project

[81] Sick City Project

[82] Tom Koch, Phd, Bioethicist, Vancouver, British Columbia, John Snow, Hero of Cholera: RIP, CMAC-JAMC –
www.ncbi.nlm.nih.gov/pmc/articles/PMC24133317/

[83] Tom Koch

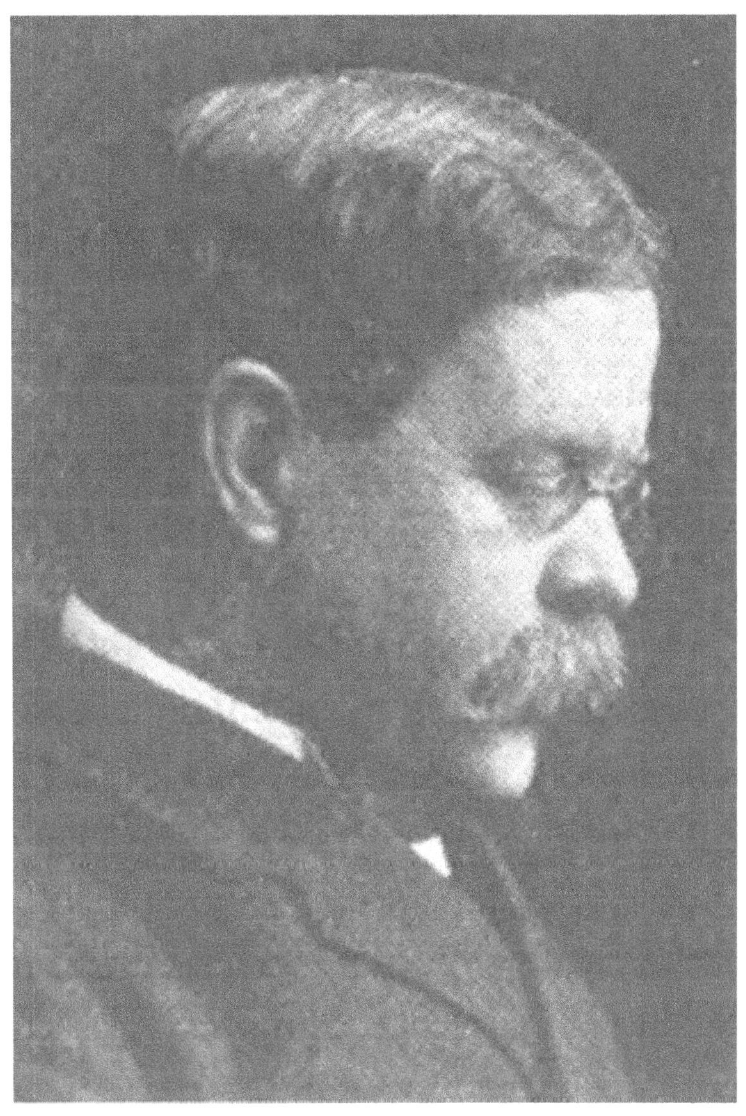

Sedgwick

Meanwhile, in England and other locations, the germ theory still had not entirely broken through by the new century. In an instance of "sour grapes," *The Lancet* continued to praise Snow's work as an anesthetist while failing to mention his breakthrough on cholera. In contrast, former critic John Simon became one of Snow's champions and finished the earlier study well after Snow's death. For his trouble, he was elevated to the top of his profession and awarded knighthood, and despite the obstinance of some, the British government was able to stem the worst of subsequent outbreaks through the fruits of Snow's research and Simon's public applications.

In a sense, Snow got the ball rolling, but it was left to Louis Pasteur and Robert Koch (1843–1910) to prove beyond doubt that microorganisms were the cause of infectious diseases such as bubonic plague, cholera, typhus, influenza, measles, and smallpox. Edward Jenner (1749–1823) had famously demonstrated that immunity to smallpox could be acquired by inoculating persons with a small quantity of cowpox, and this was in the 1760s, long before germ theory had been proved. In the 1880s, Pasteur made discoveries that led to the development of a vaccine against anthrax, leading in turn to a cascade of research that resulted in the prevention of diphtheria, mumps, measles, polio, and other morbidities. In 1897, the first vaccine for bubonic plague was developed, and 2019 saw the introduction of a vaccine against Ebola.[84] As a result, most of the microbial diseases that historically afflicted the human race have a vaccine, and plagues which used to decimate populations such as smallpox and cholera are no longer the cataclysmic threats they used to be.

There is little to no doubt in the modern day as to

---

[84] "Merck's Ervebo [Ebola Zaire Vaccine (rVSVΔG-ZEBOV-GP) live] Granted Conditional Approval in the European Union" (Press release). Merck. 11 November 2019.

Snow's excellent use of spatial analysis in the tracking of a disease's geographical progression. However, some controversy remains as to whether he fashioned his map before or after the removal of the pump, and various points of time speculation are set against the death rates by certain dates. The arc of mortality was on the downswing by the time he finished his study, and Snow was certainly not the first practitioner to establish a disease map for a specific area. Valentine Seaman fashioned an effective chart during an outbreak of yellow fever in New York near the end of the 18th century.

While Snow continues to hold his status within the medical community, he is not widely known outside of it, but that has been in part alleviated by a popular episode in the BBC series *Victoria*, starring Jenna Coleman. Professional people are often ungracious when they view their line of work depicted on screen by non-practitioners, but many medical experts believe that the series' depiction of Snow's work as anesthetist to the queen is relatively accurate. Furthermore, author Steven Johnson has produced a best-selling book on the subject with Snow as the central character while in his greatest professional crisis. A strongly researched historic novel, Johnson's work has been praised for illuminating "the intertwined histories and inter-connectedness of the spread of disease."[85] Johnson highlighted the authentic dread of those "left to tend for themselves in dark, suffocating rooms,"[86] and the vision of the dead being wheeled down the street "by the cartload."[87]

To be sure, Snow still has his detractors, many of whom evaluate his efforts through the prism of the present day. A study conducted in 2013 by the National Institutes of Health faults Snow for not adding the category of population risk and the progression of the disease over extended time to his portfolio. They note that he could have investigated common themes relevant to disparate diseases including mental health and cancer, then cross-reference them against rates of education, poverty, financial networks, crime and violence. OF course, a well-funded research organization in the absence of an outbreak can scarcely fault Snow for sticking to the disease at hand. He was not funded at all and was pursuing his investigation in the midst of an immediate crisis.

Further acts of dismissiveness came in the 1936 reprinting of *Mode of Communication of Cholera.* Wade Hampton Frost of Johns Hopkins University republished the book, selling thousands more copies than Snow ever did. However, he thought it unnecessary to include

---

[85] Goodreads, Steven Johnson's The Ghost Map: The Story of London's Most Terrifying Epidemic, and How It Changed Science, Cities, and the Modern World –www.goodreads.com/book/show/36086.The_Ghost_Map

[86] Goodreads, Steven Johnson

[87] Goodreads, Steven Johnson

Snow's London data for home visits. He listed only 23 of the 334 entries from the original document. Since Frost's effort became part of the research model for Snow's work, the error was perpetuated.

To this day, a replica of the infamous pump stands at the same intersection of Broad Street, now named Broadwick, and across the street sits the John Snow pub. At the time, having one's name bestowed on a public house was nearly as prestigious as receiving a knighthood from the reigning monarch. The replica's handle is missing, symbolizing the confirmation of Snow's theory.

Many tributes remain to Snow, who was dubbed the "most famous doctor in history" by the John Snow Society. The Society boasts over 1,000 members and is housed by the Royal Institute of Public Health in London. Each year in September, a guest is invited to present the "Pumphandle Lecture,"[88] followed by a ceremony in which a pump handle is removed.

Naturally, the successful mapping of a major disease's progression in geographic terms is much more viable today than it was over 150 years ago. Radiation victims are particularly well-armed with modern technology and can accomplish such statistical needs in a fraction of the time. Various cancers have been detected around the

---

[88] Michael A.E. Ramsay

vicinity of specific incinerators and poisonous pesticides and herbicides.

The use of geographical mapping may have brought the story of the Broad Street water pump down to students of epidemiology, and Snow is widely credited for ushering in epidemiology as a practice. However, many are surprisingly unaware of the larger statistical feat Snow managed in the "Great Experiment" conducted in South London. The visits to over 300 addresses carried a larger purpose than to gather statistics for an area measuring a few blocks. At risk of their personal health, Snow and Whiting took on the statistical realities of the entire city's water suppliers. According to Sir Austin Hill, epidemiologist and statistician, the entire breadth of Snow's accomplishment comes down to one ultimate reality: the world has been "free from epidemic cholera since the late 1800s."[89]

Above other considerations, Snow's methodology has affirmed one great truth of epidemiology. In the words of one modern practitioner, "Location and disease are inseparable."[90]

Online Resources

Other books about the plague on Amazon

---

[89] Samantha Hanja, David L. Buckeridge, James A. Hanley
[90] Dierdre Mask

Further Reading

Ball, Laura, Cholera and the Pump on Broad Street, The Life and Legacy of John Snow, *The History Teacher* Vol. 43 No. 1 (Nov., 2009) Society for History Education

Britannica.com, Cholera Through History – www.britannica.com/science/cholera/cholera-through-history

Caton, Donald, MD, John Snow's Practice of Obstetric Anesthesia, *Anesthesiology*, Jan. 2000 – www.anesthesiology.pubs.asahq.org/article.aspx?-1945835

Crosier, Scott, John Snow: The London Cholera Epidemic of 1854 – www.webprojects.oit.ncsu.edu/project/bio/83de/Black/science_reading/8.html

Douglas Laurelyn, Health and Hygiene in the Nineteenth Century. The Victorian Web, 1991 – www.victorianweb.o9rg/science/health/health10.htm

Foussianes, Victoria Mostly Got it Right, The True Story of John Snow's Cholera Breakthrough, *Town and Country Magazine*, Feb. 4, 2019

Hajna, Samantha, Buckeridge, David L., Hanley, James A., Substantiating the Impact of john Snow's

Contributions Using Data Deleted During the 1936 Reprinting of His Original Essay On the Mode of Communication of Cholera, August 26, 2015 – www.academic.oup.com/je/article/44/6/1794/2572639

History Home.UK, Cholera Comes to Britain: October 1831 – www.historyhome.co.uk/peel/p-health/cholera3.htm

Industrialization Diseases, Cholera and Great Britain – www.industrializationdiseases.wordpress.com/cholera-and-great-britain/

John Snow Society, The, About John Snow – www.honsnowsociety.org/john-snow.html

John Snow, The Father of Epidemiology, A Brief History of Public Health – www.sphweb.bumc.edu/otlt/MPH-Modules/PH/PublicHealthHistory6.html

Johnson, Alistair, John Snow and Thomas Giordani Wright, Medical Apprentices in Newcastle upon Tyne – www.kora.matrix.msu.edu/files/20/120/15-78-AE-22snow%20and%20wright%20in%20newcastle-or.pdf

Johnson, Steven, The Ghost Map: The Story of London's Most Terrifying Epidemic and How It Changed Science,

Cities, and the Modern World –
www.goodreads.com/book/show/36086.The_Ghost_Map

Koch, Tom, PhD, Bioethicist, Vancouver, British Columbia, John Snow: Hero of Cholera: RIP, CMAJ-JAMC-
www.ncbi.nlm,nih.gov/pmc/articles/PMC2412317/

Lacey, Stephen: Cholera: Calamitous Past, Ominous Future, *Clinical Infectious Diseases* Vol. 30 No. 5 (May 1995)

Mask, Dierdre, How the Father of Epidemiology Made the Connection Between Disease and Geography, Time, April 14, 2020 – www.time.com/addresses-epidemiology/

Past Medical History, John Snow and the 1854 Cholera Outbreak, Jan. 23, 2018 –
www.pastmedicalhistory.co.uk/john-snow-and-the-1854-cholera-outbreak/

PMC, U.S. National Library of Medicine, National Institutes of Health, the Mortality Rates and the Space-Time Patterns of John Snow's Cholera Epidemic Map –
www.ncbi.nlm.nih.gov/pmc/articles/PMC4521606/

Ramsay, Michael A.E., John Snow, MD: Anesthetist to the Queen of England and Pioneer Epidemiologist, Bay7lor University Medical Center (Jan. 2006) –
www.nchi.nih.gov/pmc/articles/PMC135279

Sandler, Dale P., John Snow and modern-Day Epidemiology, July 1, 2000, American Journal of Epidemiology – www.academi.oup.com/aje/article/152/1/1/139141

Science Museum, Brought to Life, Cholera Comes to Victorian London – www.broughttolife.sciencemuseum.org.uk/broughttolife/themes/publichealth/cholera

Sick City Project, John Snow and Cholera – www.sickcityproject.wordpress.com/2013/03/11/john-snow-and-cholera/

The Social Historian, Death in the Time of Cholera – www.thesocialhistorian.com/death-time-cholera

Tuthill, Kathleen, UCLA Department of Epidemiology, Fielding School of Public Health, John Snow and the Broad Street Pump, On the Trail of an Epidemic, Nov., 2003 – www.ph.ucla.edu/epi/snowcricketarticle.html

UCLA Department of Epidemiology, Cholera, Brief History During the Snow Era – www.ph.ucla.edu/snow3/1859maps/cholera_prevailingtheories_a2.html

UCLA Department of Epidemiology – www.ph.ucla.edu/epi/snow/victoria.html

Vachon, David, UCLA, John Snow Blames Water Pollution for Cholera Epidemic, UCLA, Part One, UCLA Department of Epidemiology – www.ph.ucla.edu/epi/snow/fatherofepidemiology.html

Waters, Ralph M., John Snow, First Anesthetist, *Bios,* Vol. 17 no 1 (March 1936) Beta Beta Beta Biological Society

Wills, Matthew, John Snow and the Birth of Epidemiology, Daily Jstor.org, May 28, 2018 – www.daily.jstor.org/john-snow-and-the-birth-of-epidemiology/

Zielinski, Sarah, John Snow and the Grand Experiment, Smithsonian Magazine, August 18, 2010 – www.smithsonianmag.com/science-nature/cholera-john-snow-and-the-grand-experiment-3349689/

Free Books by Charles River Editors

Discounted Books by Charles River Editors

We have titles at a discount price of just 99 cents everyday. To see which of our titles are currently 99 cents, click on this link.